My Journey of Yoga

A Quest within

Akshay R

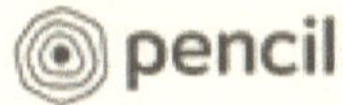

ISBN 978-93-5610-576-8

Published in India 2022 by Pencil

A brand of
One Point Six Technologies Pvt. Ltd.
123, Building J2, Shram Seva Premises,
Wadala Truck Terminal, Wadala (E)
Mumbai 400037, Maharashtra, INDIA
E connect@thepencilapp.com
W www.thepencilapp.com

Author biography

Budding as a young writer,the author has tried bringing about sharing his views regarding what yoga is actually about.He has been practising yoga from 5 years by now and also being a junior doctor in the field of Yoga and Naturopathy.He has completed his studies from SDM College of Naturopathy and Yogic Sciences,a pioneer institution in the field of Yoga and Naturopathy. Suffocated world with lots of western culture and lifestyle ,there is a need for the reforming this materialism with the ancient wisdom what our ancients have left for us.With this intention the author has tried sharing his views and interests what changes need to be made in the society by encorporating yoga in their lives.Change always comes from within,Be the change you want to see in the society.And hence for this change to be seen within and henceforth in the society it requires imbibing yoga in our lives.The author has taken so much of work in shaping out this book so that it comes out in a good manner for the readers of present generation.Hope this book could bring about changes in the lives of readers and the message of yoga is spread all over.

CONTENTS

LIGHT OF TRUTH 9

AN INSIGHT INTO INDIAN HISTORY 11

NATIONAL INTEGRITY THE PILLAR OF NATION 14

INTRODUCTION TO YOGA 16

YOGA AN INTEGRAL PART OF INTEGRITY 19

THE STORY OF SHABARI 21

THE ESSENCE OF SPIRITUALITY IN YOGA 23

DESIRE-THE DAY IT WAS BORN!! 25

QUANTUM THEORY OF YOGA 27

THE STORY OF RAMAKRISHNA PARAMAHAMSA 29

TEACHINGS FROM OUR SCRIPTURES 31

THE STORY OF ADAM AND EVE 33

TEACHINGS FROM THE SCRIPTURES 35

THE KEY TO KARMA 37

THE STORY OF KARMA 39

THE KEY TO BHAKTHI 41

THE STORY OF BHAKTHI 43

THE KEY TO JNANA 45

THE STORY OF JNANA 47

FROM THE CONCENTRATION CAMPS 49
LIFE IN CONCENTRATION CAMPS 51
YOGA AND EXISTENTIALISM 55
THE ORIGIN OF YOGA 60
THE PRACTICE OF YOGA 63
A NOTE ON PATANJALI YOGA 65
A NOTE ON PATHANJALI YOGA 71
A NOTE ON HATHA YOGA -1 73
A NOTE ON HATHA YOGA -2 76
A NOTE ON HATHA YOGA -3 79
A NOTE ON HATHA YOGA-4 82
BEYOND THE "I" 86
PANCHAKOSHA CONCEPT OF YOGA
IN THERAPY 90
YOGA AS A THERAPY 94
THE THEORY OF CAUSE AND EFFECT 96
THE ESSENCE OF GITA 99
THE STORY OF GOOD PUNYA 102
RELAXATION TECHNIQUES 104
THE MESSAGE OF SWAMI VIVEKANANDA 106
WHY ONE NEEDS TO CHANT AUM 111
OMKARA MEDITATION 119
YOGA NIDRA 123
ZEN MEDITATION 128

NADHANUSANDANA 134
VIPASSANA MEDITATION 137
TRANSCEDENTAL MEDITATION 141
INSTANT RELAXATION TECHNIQUE(IRT) 143
QUICK RELAXATION TECHNIQUE(QRT) 146
DEEP RELAXATION TECHNIQUE(DRT) 148
CYCLIC MEDITATION 151
PRANIC ENERGISATION TECHNIQUE(PET) 155
MIND SOUND RESONANCE TECHNIQUE(MSRT) 159
MASTERING THE EMOTIONS TECHNIQUE(MEMT) 164
MIND IMAGERY TECHNIQUE(MIRT) 169
VIJNANA SADHANA KAUSALAM(VISAK) 174
ANANDA AMRTA SINCHANA(ANAMS) 179
THE FIVE VAYUS 186
THE MYSTERY OF DEATH 191
WHY DO YOGIS SAY NAMASTE 196

Preface

As millions of you have different views regarding what actually yoga is in this modern world, this book out here penned down by me goes on explaining the views which was brought forth infront of me while learning yoga. I have tried explaining the forefront view of our nation's culture and how yoga has been able to groom it and it's necessity in our today's world!!

Hope this book of mine would give you a clear view and help you in taking up yoga!!I have just forefronted my view about my experiences through yoga with all my eorts!!I am greatful to all the readers out there for taking a look into my first book.Though very young at age, I have taken all my eorts in making this book look interesting.I am also thankful to all the teachers throughout my life till here who have made me understand what our Indian culture is all about.

I hope you would love the journey through the world of yoga brought out by me here.

With regards
Akshay Ravikumar

Introduction

Marking so many changes in today's world we are witnessing so many transformations. Be it good or bad we are changing in a way what Dr.Abdul kalam once said that India would be a super power by the end of 2020. We are marching towards the new era of so called "global power". But what wondered me is how far is India being different from the rest of world. There are lot of aspects which we all should look upon from spirituality,secularism to being one of the biggest democracies of the world. But there is a lot more we have to see through when it comes to Indian history. Back from days of Indus valley civilization from where they typically say India derived it's name we have got a vast history which would take us a lot of our lives to just look

back and we would realise it's more vast than what we have actually thought of.

More rather I feel comfortable in calling India as "Bharat"as it gives me so much pride in doing so because that's where my writings further are going through all about.

In sanskrit, "Bha" Means "light" And "rat" Means "one who has devoted his or her entire life in search of that".This one word seems to tell a lot about India and our present lives. We surely are in search of this light of truth!!

LIGHT OF TRUTH

So what's this light of truth which I was speaking all about!!
You may wonder about the divine light which we may have come across in movies when a person dies.A flame like light actually is shown travelling upwards and suddenly vanishing!! Seems so nice but it's actually depicted in movies to convey the fact that the soul is leaving the body. The light which now I am speaking about is entirely different from this view of movies.Its the light which comes through having continous insight of oneself. So why is this insight essential? Is it really needed for existence? We have been living all through ourlives reaching with all our desires. What makes us necessary to go in search of this light? This surely would be each and everyone's question out there. Surely even I used to wonder as a while ago since my childhood.Similar to as a child how Narendra used to wander in search of a person who would answer his question regarding God even I used to look out for all these answers.Still in the same search though but I was able to unleash a lotof things in this journey of mine through a lot of sources may be people or books or from personalities of our history.Yoga at sometime also helped me in experiencing this light of truth at many instances which I can say even many yogic practitioners might have experienced.This light of truth is

what explains you in understanding the purpose of life surely what everyone want to know of!! But before explaining about this light of truth I would go on with many of the aspects of what India has seen through so far and why yoga has been a necessity in these aspects.

AN INSIGHT INTO INDIAN HISTORY

May sound typical but for sure I was a kind of student who never looked upon history during my school daysas an essential subject. As what difference could it bring after all! We can't go back and change it and why is it so much important to study some ruler and his reforms after all!!Anyways now we can't do anything with it greatly as we have acccepted and living through democracy.We are living on the lines of "King is for the people, of the people and by the people"!! But these views of me changed as in a while as I was coming across a book by Dr.Anupama Niranjana.History surely has a role in shaping our present and future dream on "Bhavya Bharat nirman" Project. India, the land of holy ganga river,The land where Hinduism has deep roots through it,The land where all religions are followed,the land of purity and so on.. India has been also referred to as Aryavartha,jambudweepa,bharathakhanda and so on. 'Aryavartha', as first land terrestrials lived here known as'Aryans'.'Jambudweepa'because of the 'jambu'fruit which was grown in India over ages ago.Moreover Indian land has been referred in our Indian history as "good collector".We have seen all the essence of many religions absorbed into this beautiful land.They say whatever be the severity of flood, the water gets absorbed into this land.Such beauty is our Bharat!! Going on,Our Indian land was ruled by one of the greatest ruler by name Bharatha!! Probably the best king of all times because Indian land flourished to a lot during his time!!Later the best kings probably would be Harshavardhana and Ashoka. They are called as best kings not for the fact that they had a very big empire and due to their winning streaks on neighbouring lands but because of the reforms they brought about and the way of caretaking their subjects make them immensely great. Indeed there was a lot of fights within ourselvelves later whether as a mark of pride or due to the hatredness towards one another fostering the foreign rulers to our country.The first example for this was the incoming of Alexander the great, though he had a big army he was strongly resisted by a brave woman cleophis of massaga who with just 30,000 soldiers resisted the army of greeks which had fourfold of this strength. Though she lost the battle but what ensued was the heavy loss of Greek soldiers and Alexander had to return back. After all this scene of bravery what followed was the fights within ourselves. The fight between the Rajputs, Yadavas made it all for the foreign rulers to enter India and established their sovereignty. Among those foreigners, rulers like Mohammad ghazni came to India 16 times and looted the wealth taking it to his homeland. Another would be Mohammad ghori who not only looted but also destroyed many temples and beautiful shrines.Though some of the rulers resisted, they had their own relatives who helped the foreign rulers. One such example was Prithviraj chauhan who strongly resisted but his own father in law joined hands with Mohammad ghori. The southern kings were no less for this! The Pandyas, Cheras, Cholas, Pallavas of kanchi, Hoysalas were all the same. This made an opportunity for minister of Allauddin khilji, Malik kafar to easily capture all these and destroy these kingdoms.Later we have seen the establishment of Portuguese, Dutch, French, and finally the Britishers estabilish their rule. They took the mere advantage of this hatredness within us in slowly raising for the power and making us live in the black shadow of slavery. But going through all these what have we actually lost?Surely it's the strength of unitywhich we all were supposed to depict at these times.We may call it as "National integrity" in other words.

NATIONAL INTEGRITY THE PILLAR OF NATION

Ahead later after Independence we saw a bright future waiting for us. As Pandit Jawaharlal Nehru said on 14th August 1947 midnight,"When the whole world is sleeping, India is rising to a bright future ahead! A March towards a new destiny of hope! One generation has ended,a new one is coming up and the fact of offering oneself for the nation and it's people should be instilled deep within it.Great words indeed!!

Marking his words in this new generation,are we in such offerring is the question? Surely this offering of oneself is also in need for this integrity. One more thing what made the whole world look towards India was humanity. Amid all these threats and challenges we have been able to support one another and have welcomed all the outsiders with love and peace.This probably could be because of our culture and spirituality of course!! But what really has put threat tous of course is our continuation of slavery!! Slavery to what? Nothing but to our own greeds, The need that only 'I' should flourish no matter what happens with the rest of the society. This thought surely will end in nowhere but fights like in past history. This fight would be probably not only with the society around but also within ourselves this time!! Probably that's what our elders speak

about saying the next world war would not be for money or pride but for the basic amenities and also to estabilish our own
inner peace. And of course we are seeing those signs at present times!! We must also wonder what better world are we gifting to our next generation?We would boast about technology and Science to our future generation but at the cost of what?? We are losing alot of the values of ecosystem in doing so!! One must think about these things as it's the duty of every person in this regard.Surely if science would have been progressed in such a way that man would have been less possessive and greedy as of now all our scientic works would have got more meaning and worth to be looked!!

INTRODUCTION TO YOGA

Walking on the paths of our ancient sages who gave us this very own gift, Yoga. So what is actually yoga??
Probably my favourite definition would be 'Yujyathe anena ithi yogaha".Yoga is the one essential science which
brings about union between the body and mind as it has been said in texts. So going on further what's this union all about?Why is it needed? So why is it being acknowledged and internationally propagated so much!! This question truly makes a sense for a beginner in the practice of yoga. Yoga is not just union of body and mind but also it's the one aspect which makes us to come together.It unites people to harmoniously interact with each other. The very basic aspect of yoga is to bring down our desires or in clear view our greed or attachments. Maybe everyone can't get bliss at sametime in yoga but surely would feel some changes in their path. Yoga according to the founder Patanjali maharshi is said as "yogas chitta vritti nirodhah" meaning as complete cessation of thoughts.Many of you would ask me ,why do we need to obstruct thoughts ?As Einstein says thinking and imagination are the ones needed for man to do something really great. Man has been referred to as rational animal and superior to others because of his power of thinking and humanity. Then why do we need to obstruct thoughts? It's nothing but stilling

the unwanted fluctuations.We all would have seen a pond so calm.It seems so beautiful to see this scenic view more probably during evening times during sunset. But what does it happen when we throw a stone to it?There is surely a lot of disturbance in the form of ripples or waves!! But later after some time if there is a calm environment, it again becomes still. Samething happens with our mind indeed, the stone whatever I was referring to was nothing but the 'thoughts' and the one which creates this 'calm environment' is nothing else than the practise of "Yoga". So with this example I guess one would get a complete view of what yoga could do actually. We must also understand that yoga isn't just a philosophy or practice, more than that it's a science. As in our view what science actually aims for is to search for the truth. Maybe we do it by research and try to find the truth out by so called inventions or discoveries. Even Yoga does the same thing.We are just discovering ourselves,the inner truth residing within ourselves. Another classical definition about yoga would be the one given by Swami Vivekananda. He says yoga as a means of reducing one's own evolution to a single life of very few months or days or to few minutes. Probably this is what even Shankaracharya goes on telling about in his work bhajagovindam.

"Punarapi jananam punarapi maranam punarapi janani jatare
shayanam. Iha samsare bahudoostare kripaya paare pahi murare"

He asks God to relieve him from this clutches of birth-death cycle. And that's what Yoga can do at!! Many of you would then question me why should we get relieved from this birth and death cycle? I mean like I am so happy, wealthy and with all the needs whichever I want!! Then why should I not ask for rebirth??

I have tried to find an answer for these questions in the next chapters as you go on.

YOGA AN INTEGRAL PART OF INTEGRITY

Maybe these words would make you bit confusing as such!! But truly it's one aspect what yoga can achieve if driven in right direction!! "Integral" means"part of a whole" And integrity surely would mean doing the right thing at right time probably by being together in a large community. Yoga is that part of whole of this Integrity of a community which brings one together to do the right thing.This is what is very much essential for a nation to build upon in a progressive manner!! Indeed the Varna system has got us in various terms of inequality in the society posing a threat to the development of the nation!! And even the money mindedness in people in this rat race has got us to think of only about oneself. We are going towards the fact to accumulate more and more merely thinking about others. No matter what happens to others or nation only I should prosper. This is the one cause why still our several regions of India is still seen with poverty amidst it's development. Yoga could actually act as a powerful tool in fighting this 'pandemic'.The reason to call this as as pandemic because of the widespread thought of greed among all of us.We need to revive the thought of caring for others rather caring for oneself all the time!! Now the question would be how? The answer would be in yoga itself which always stresses upon to give away with our desires. Nothing is permanent. We come and we go and all that we percieve are just momentary in this physical world . We would probably see this in one of the stories of Ramayana!!

THE STORY OF SHABARI

We all would have heard about Ramayana from our childhood.This great epic has been worshipped from
ages because it's the story of maryada purushottama Sri Rama. Now you would also been heard of Shabari.
The devotion she had towards the great Lord himself Sri Rama.Now I have shared my yogic views through it as you go on with the story. Shabari who was a great devotee of Sri Rama used to wait for him for so many years. Daily she used to pluck fruits for him and wait for him! Though she was so much aged she never got fed up waiting for Rama.She used to always wait for him calling Rama, Rama!! Then one final day she was able to meet
him without knowing that they were actually Rama and lakshmana when these duo went to shabari's hut with hunger seeking food and shelter. She fed the fruits she had and gave them shelter.
Later did she come to know that the person was none other than Rama himself. Very much pleased by her devotion Rama asks her as what she wished for? He said that whatever it is she would ask for would be granted. He asked her whether she wanted to be free from her old age and become young again? Or she wished for lots of wealth? And so on. But shabari refused to all of these!! Then finally Rama asked her what she wanted from him. Then Shabari went on further saying, "Hey Lord,

everything in this world is as minutely impermanent as the bubble on the water.Whatever you asked me the wealth,young age is all temporary. What I want is a permanent freedom from this life of birth and death. And that sure permanent place would be reaching to your divine feet. Please bless me to be in your divine abode!! A nice story indeed to be read!! But what matters is her words of immaterialism about the world!! She waited all through her life for Rama with so much patience and devotion and when asked for any boon she could have asked for many stuffs what we in her place would prefer for!! But she relented as she was aware that this world was just momentary. Her truth of life was to serve
and meet Rama and when she met him her life truth had been discovered and there was not any thing now essential for her.This story surely teaches us to give away our materialistic desires and aspire for the Divine truth within ourselves.Definitely yoga and spirituality could do a lot in unleashing this truth within ourselves!!

THE ESSENCE OF SPIRITUALITY IN YOGA

Now basically let's understand what's spirituality is all about before moving forward with my topic above.
"Spirituality" basically comes from the Latin word "spiron" meaning "the breath' or " to breathe". And they say the day our first breath started I mean our birth there itself originated our spirituality.So you may ask me whether are we all having spirituality within us!! Yes of course but the only thing is we still haven't discovered it!! Then the question is how to discover it? Exactly the one and only way may be Yoga. Because it's the only path wherein you are focussing on yourself. Spirituality and devotion according to me are entirely different.Because devotion maybe seen as different perspectives in different sectors and religions. One example is the way we worship God like some worship linga or the moorthi what we say, but some see the same devotion with their work as Basavanna,renowned saint says "kayakave kailasa" and many would also express their devotion by religious fasting as we see in cases of Muslims during ramzan, by doing certain number of circumambulation to God in temples.All these are truly good for a person who is in the divine path of God. But in the case of spirituality it is attributed as same thing in all the religions. That is

understanding the very own cause of your breath into this world. I mean the cause for your existence. This is the one beauty of spirituality as it can never be religious as in cases of today's science but it is always truth-seeking.When you actually understand this truth you start loving everyone around you in this world no matter whether he has done good or bad to you. The basic principle that all the religious texts nomatter the Bhagavadgita or Quran or The holy Bible have said the same thing, To love one and all !! But in our today's society without knowing this truth we so called educationists are fighting in the name of religions instead of accepting one another and live in harmony which could actually help in our nation's progress. I guess Yoga could help you all to understand this truth as it brings forth the concept of "Union".That is the reason maybe most of the nation's have internationally accepted Yoga and have started following it.For sure the whole world started praising India and saw what is India when we gifted this Yoga to the entire world through International yoga day on 21st June every year. And we have seen the power of its influence all across the globe on this day.

DESIRE-THE DAY IT WAS BORN!!

So when was all our desires born!! One would say when I became matured, or when I saw a chocolate, when I saw a lamborghini or an audi car and so on…..In one of the recent books I was coming across this view which says that the source of all the desires origins right from the time when a child is born.The child in mother's womb feels that it owns the right of it. But it's actually not the womb it owns but just the shelter offered by the womb.Later when the child grows and mother starts to feed the child,the child feels that he owns his mother….. But actually only the act of feeding or getting nutrition from mother is owned by the child and not his mother itself. These misconceptions which begins here; goes on and on and the desire that everything it sees in the society is felt as if he has owned it which results in the craving. In all these the point I want to show here is that the karma i.e.,the action of getting nutrition and shelter derived from the mother is the right of the child but the womb of mother doesn't belong to him.Same thing moving on over it's age as the child gets older and older he should feel that karma is just his right but the karmaphala or the fruits of work is always decided by the God himself. If we understand this truth surely there would be no greed and rat race in the society. As a coincidence or by chance I don't know both spirituality and this greed of individuals begins at the same time that is at the time of birth. The one that decides which one would the child accepts in these two depends upon by the fact of the karma the child adopts to in its later life as well as the karmas of its previous birth!! So coming to Yoga how can yoga help in reducing these desires which has come from over years or from many of our births!! The answer would be detachment.As one goes on with the practice of yoga, all these actions and their sources starts declining. One feels detached towards all these materialistic stuffs and goes in search of his own inner self, from the conscious world to an inner subconscious world which resides deep inside oneself.

QUANTUM THEORY OF YOGA

Recently I was coming across a discovery that there are more minute particles than the electrons and protons
known as Leptoquarks. This wondered me so much as the term "atom" itself is so much small and electron even more smaller,probably the most minutest one.Then imagine about leptoquarks.Then what wondered to me even more was the theory that all these leptoquarks are the same in every individual.

May be the electrons would differ but the leptoquarks were the same in every individual. So it would mean that all the individuals were the same. But it is we who have differed among ourselves by making various grades in the society. We are all the one and the same deep within our compostiton that is in this aspect of leptoquarks. Probably both living and non living things are the same but what makes different is the thing called
"life".After our death even we would lose all our identity. You could have experienced this instance at the time of funeral. No one will call him by person but mostly refer with the term " body".This is life!!

Many times we also behave as non living things even though we are alive. You may ask me how and when? The answer would be when we lose our humanity.There are a lot of instances wherein we have seen people losing this very basic character not only towards others but also towards themselves.Many great men and authors refer this kind of race of humans as animals. But I would rather call them as non living objects. Because there are a lot of instances where animals have shown humanity. Now let me come to yogic point of view, last year I came across a concept wherein the people who were teachers of transcedental meditation said in one of the classes that this meditation has a lot of effects on leptoquarks very much signicantly and the effect or impact would be different among people based on their practice and severity.They had also shown many of their results after the practise to propound this effects. Thus this made one thing clear that yoga has a lot of effects on the quantum level indeed.In today's world wherein "quantum theory" is gaining importance in every field including our modern medical field, the science of yoga is no exception for this.The only thing is that one needs to discover for himself by practice!!

THE STORY OF RAMAKRISHNA PARAMAHAMSA

So giving away with all desires how should our path be? I mean how should our sadhana be?? Let's move on with a story before I explain about these aspects. Once Sri Ramakrishna paramahamsa was meditating on the banks of river Kali. The river was so calm and peaceful with the birds chirping around and a cool breeze with quite pleasant nature around. On the other side of the river he could see a saint performing severe penance to please Lord shiva. This holy man used to perform most strict penance everyday sitting with utmost concentration and worship to please the God. Everyday Ramakrishna paramahamsa used to watch his strict penance on the other side of the river. One fine day the God pleased by his penance came infront of him and blessed this man with great powers,which in yogic terms what we call as "siddhi".This holy man became very much proud and arrogant that he had been blessed with super powers by God and had got a boon.He then started to walk on the water with his power and came towards Sri Ramakrishna paramahamsa. Then feeling so much proud about himself he said, "Did you see my powers now. I have been blessed by God with these powers. And I am still seeing you meditating on something from so many days. What are you doing? I think you are just wasting time without anything to ask for and just simply meditating. ".Sri Ramakrishna parmahamsa replied to him, " I think you wasted all your efforts of penance!!".The holy man became furious," You are jealous seeing my powers. How could you say that all my tapas became useless. See my powers here. I came walking on the water from the other side of river till here. Could you have done that?".Then Sri Ramakrishna paramahamsa just smiled and replied to him, "Probably I can't do that. But I could exactly say one thing that you wasted all your efforts. You could have probably just given a coin to the boatman out there and he could have made you cross the river till here from the other side. But you spent all these years for these powers and all that you did was just to cross a river". Hearing these words the holy man's pride came all the way down and he fell at Sri Ramakrishna paramahamsa's feet and asked for his forgiveness. What a beautiful story indeed!! But what is the message that we get from this story is all that matters the most! The goal which the holy man had is indeed not worth of!! Whenever we are in any form of sadhana, our grail should be towards truth and in search of this,we may acquire a lot of powers as the holy man got; but, all these powers should never be one's desire or the goal of one's practice. In yoga we refer this as siddhi.Even if we get these powers as a result of our practice or sadhana these should never be misused and if at all if we need to use, it should be reserved only for the service of mankind or for helping others who are at difficulties.We should never become arrogant about these powers and be in a dilemma thinking that this is the ultimate goal of one's practice. As I already said science should always go in search of truth and so is yoga!!

TEACHINGS FROM OUR SCRIPTURES

When anyone goes on with our scriptures,We find a lot of instances which tell us what actually life is all about!

Not only this,every scripture has seen the God as a same form!! That is a source of energy making this cycle of universe to work upon.This energy is indeed infinite like the sun wherein we see the infinite fusion reactions going on and on.How has been yoga and spirituality seen in our scriptures?This would also probably would be the questions from the point of view of many philosophers and yoga believers. There are a lot of views about yoga in Hinduism as we are the ones who have accepted polytheism. Hence we have always been in discussions,opinions and research from our practice to everything in our worship.Even in our Hindu texts we find a lot of views regarding yogic concepts and I feel you all would agree with that.

But what matters among all these is the essence. All these scriptures and these holy people ask to accept the ultimate truth that can happen only by finding out your meaning of existence.

In theist Hinduism and books we see yoga as a means to become closer to God may be in the form of karma, bhakthi and jnana yoga as explained in

Srimadbhagavadgitha. But the path which one chooses depends on one's own intention and desires.And I feel that for the other two, karma yoga would be very much essential for a normal man. Because without work you can't do the other in today's world.You may ask me that I am a teacher and I am able to work only with my jnana and how could you say karma yoga is essential for me? The answer is even when you wanted to earn the jnana you should have done some karma or in other terms work as nothing comes free of cost in this world. If it comes freely then surely there is something to be questioned about at! Even the yogis who gain the divine knowledge, I mean jnana should have done some karma in the form of tapas or penance for that.That's what even Basavanna says as "Work is worship" asking people to accept their own duties or work as a form of worship. Here also we would see karma yoga as the source for Bhakthi yoga. This was just my view and I don't know how far you people would accept it. Now as I feel that I have been a lot awhile with Hindu scriptures, I feel to move forward with scriptures of other religions. But before that, I would like to go on with one nice story in my next chapter !!

THE STORY OF ADAM AND EVE

The story which I am now speaking to you about can be found in both the books I.e., Bible as well as Quran. This is a nice story which maybe many of us might have heard. God in the process of creation created two first human beings out known as Adam and Eve.Adam was created from the dust whereas Eve has been said to be created from the rib of Adam. According to the myth these duo were the first man and woman. These two

were on the belief that humanity is an essence of a single family and we all have descended the law of humanity from these beings. These two were placed in the Garden of Eden and were asked to look after it. They were allowed to eat fruits from any of the trees except from two trees. They were potentially very

pure souls.All went on quite well and they were living happily and never went to eat fruits from the forbidden two trees out of the fear of being punished. But once a wicked serpant came to the garden. In Islamic books they call it as sataan. This wicked serpant persuaded the duo to have the fruit from the first tree,The tree of knowledge of good and evil. And this made them to do destructive concepts which were evil.God then curses the serpant to ground. And that's why serpant is said to walk on its belly even today. Then these two were informed by God about the consequences of disobeying them and they were thus prevented from having fruit from the second tree, that is the tree of life, which would give them immortality. Then he curses them for their sin and expels them from the garden of Eden.And these descendants of Adam and Eve are we "human beings".These two out of their greed committed the sin of eating fruits what was forbidden from them by God. And hence the birth of man itself is a sin according to this story. All our spiritual and yogic practices are the need for us to come out of the bondage of this sin. We can do that only when we introspect ourselves through yoga and bring down our desires which is the cause of all sufferings.

TEACHINGS FROM THE SCRIPTURES

Now having views about Bhagavadgitha let's move on to other scriptures, the holy Bible and Quran. Bible, the holy book of Christianity has spoken a lot about love and non-violence. Love for one another and love to see everyone as one.In one of the Christian literature, I was finding Jesus writings wherein he says,"I and my father are one".We find this same concept in yoga as union."Yogas chitta vritti nirodhaha", when you cease to identify the fluctuations of mind there is yoga, identification of self bringing about union. The principle of unity is brought out here. That can only happen through love for everyone and oneself which is what said in both gospels as well as our Patanjali yoga books. Love not violence is the only way to truth.We have to live as wholeness with the nature which is all being spoken even in yoga to understand the reality of nature and it's existence. The second concept brought out here is nonviolence. As you have seen some of the Christians and their speeches, they consider everyone as the children of God and no one should be harmed in order to be closer to God. We can find the similar concept in yoga wherein Patanjali says Ahimsa is the only way to develop compassion,
"Ahimsa prathishtayam tatsannidau vaira tyagah".

The compassion which develops leads us in identifying oneself with others giving rise to oneness with nature, same thing is what has been said even in Bible. Whether Bible or Quran or Bhagavadgita all have preached the same thing i.e., to be united with love and compassion for one another. It's just our ego which comes as a barrier in this act of accepting one another to live in harmony.We usually pray for God for many of our needs but how many of us actually care or pray for the welfare of God who gives everything we ask for to us.If God is happy the whole world would be happy.Even if anyone is sad,he would make them happy.But just imagine if he goes into the shadow of dukha or sadness.Everything around us would come to a halt.All these scriptures were written to give the message of unity to explain how the laws of nature would work.With this thought in mind let's give equal importance to the essence of all religions in our day to day lives.Let us inculcate the message of yoga what has been said in every holy scriptures in our day to day lives.

THE KEY TO KARMA

We have heard some lessons from our ancient Upanishads as "shareera madhyamam khalu dharma sadhanam" This shareera or the body is vehicle for which we all should act. For any being we don't have a good body or a bad body as such. This vehicle or the body's performance or state is maintained by the karma or action which

we do. And how well we take care of this body is only through our actions. And exactly as upanishads say this shareera is a form through which we can follow the path of dharma which allows atma or soul to reach its destination. That is what even in kathopanishad it's mentioned by yama to nachiketa as such,

"Atmanam rathinam viddhi
shareeram rathameva thu
buddhim thu sarathim viddhi
manah pragraha mevacha indriyani
hayanahurvishayansteshugocharan
atmendriyamanoyuktam bhoktetyahurmaneeshinaha"

I am fortunate enough that I remember some of my lessons from my school days of the kathopanishad. So atma is called the controller of the chariot, the charioteer. The buddhi is it's driver and mind is the rope or reins of horses.The indriyas are the horses which pull the chariot.The atma enjoys the worldly pleasures through indriyas or the horses and the vehicle or the mode is the chariot or the body.

So we have seen people saying he is doing good work or he is doing bad work. So does it mean that karma is divided into good or bad. Not surely because karma itself is neither good nor bad.It is the motive which makes the karma to be good or bad. Let's take an example for this!! A knife in the hands of a doctor who is piercing and doing an operation and imagine the patient dies. So can we call his karma bad? Not at all, because his motive was not to kill the patient but overall his motive was to save the patient's life. Imagine the same knife in the hands of a serial killer, and he pierces and the person dies. Surely he would be called as a bad man and his karma would be called as destructive. So in these two cases karma is the same, they are piercing the body with a knife, but one to save the life and the other to take it out. So karma itself can never be called as good or bad but it depends only on the motive through which it is always done. Then you may ask me should we expect the fruits? Not at all,we should never think to have the fruit of mango tree just because we watered it daily. Even the tree never has its own fruits, but has it served for the others and relieves their hunger pangs.We should do a karma with good motive but the end result should never be governed by us. It should be left to the Almighty above. Whether he wishes to give the fruit as sweet or bitter, everything depends on him! We are just the means of performing the karma with a motive to serve the mankind or the existence around.

THE STORY OF KARMA

I don't know how many of you have actually heard this story.Probably we all would have heard mahabharatha only till the pandavas getting back their kingdom but never later. So followed by the mahabharatha war, the pandavas got back their kingdom. Sri krishna renounced his kingdom and later went to forest and was sleeping near a tree.A hunter by name jara mistook Sri krishna's leg to be that of an animal and accidently shot
an arrow. Feared about the consequences of krishna's anger he asked Sri krishna for his forgiveness. But even in the death bed, Sri krishna understood the cause of this incident and forgave the hunter and never became angry.He blessed the hunter and left for his divine abode. Now what was the cause of death that
Sri krishna had understood?? It was due to karmas of his previous birth which had been accounted in the form of samskaras. Sri krishna in his previous birth as Sri Rama in tretha yuga had killed vali with an arrow when he was fighting with sugreeva.Violating the rule of war nomatter for what purpose it was done, it was a sin and vali again was reborn as hunter and had shot arrow on Sri krishna. This is what we say as karma hits back. Though Sri Rama had done the action for a good purpose but in doing so he his violation accounted him for the cause of karma.This story indeed tells us how powerful karma is!!Even the Lord

himself was not spared from the bondage of karma and he had to face through it!! The greatest Dharmaraja, who was said to be the avatar of yama himself had to be a while in hell because of one small sin of telling lie to drona in the mahabharatha war.This is what is known as Universal truth of nature ,we all are the part of nature and not creators. We should indeed start going on following with the laws of nature and understand it's existential philosophy through yogic practices.

THE KEY TO BHAKTHI

I was recently coming across a video of sadhu who was standing in one leg for over years in himalayas even during heavy rain.This sadhu was meditating for very long hours on God.

Basically I was wondering what kept this sadhu keep on going with his practice even in such difficult condition that too with one leg!!My father who has visited these himalayas everytime used to tell me how these sadhus keep on going with their sadhana.And one of the magical beauty of himalayas is that it's a place where in you would fall in love with nature and nothing else, no material wishes would exist. These sadhus have nothing to wish for and all the way they are in their own world searching for the truth of their existence. What has kept them going? It is with no doubt the bhakthi or faith!! It's faith in the creation of this universe, may call it as God in terms of a theist.Their way of practices maybe different. But all of them are exactly in search of the supreme source behind this world. In my lectures I was always told about bhakthi as intense devotion to God. Nothing but "saa thasmin parama prema roopa" as said in Narada bhakthi sutra. Devotion to God has been said as intense personification of the love towards him. It's compared to the sweetness of a nectar. And one's bhakthi in the practice of yoga should always be continous like an oil pouring from one vessel to another. One who has instilled this bhakthi always feels contended, perfect and immortal. He will become truptha. These won't allow him to have any desires except for the God. Now basically how can one develop bhakthi or what is the

main quality needed? It is humility because even God himself is humble enough and likes those people with the same quality.We all are in the arrogance which shankaracharya refers to as" moodajana", in the pride that we are the rulers of this universe.This pride or ego has what made us to lose faith in God. A bhaktha should always surrender to God with extreme humility in order to go through the divine path of bhakthi. Though the goal

of bhakthi is same, it has different paths when it comes with practice by different religions. And yoga is the one which acts like a cord in tieing all these cords or paths. Thus it strengthens the cord by holding it tightly and allowing oneself to reach it easily without any breaks or obstacles. Thus yoga should never be seen as religious and should always be seen as a means of entity to surrender oneself in the service of God in all the religions. Then there would be probably a meaning to each one of our lives in saving the humankind by avoiding conflicts in the name of religions. That's what yoga says, Love the divine soul in each and every individual, if u can't then you probably can't see the divine God even when he stands in front of you!!

THE STORY OF BHAKTHI

Once a child was born to a brahmin unwed mother.Then she left him abandoned in a basket oating in the river ganga. Later a Muslim Weaver who saw a child floating near the banks of ganga picked him up and raised him. The child was named Kabir. 'Kabir' means 'The servant of God'.As name suggests he was so much lled with bhakthi in Lord and used to ask his teachers such probing questions that would make them difficult to answer. The teachers got angry and drove him out of the school. Though he was brought up as a Muslim he accepted the truth in both the religions. He was always engaged in search of true knowledge and complete detachment. Jnana teaches him,"Brahma satyam,jagat midhya" and vairagya teaches oneself to detach from the world when one learns this basic principle of life. And Kabir was no less in imbibing these two qualities. His quest for knowledge was so much that he did not leave any religious scriptures untouched. He read Quran, Hindu sastras,su saint lectures and so on. Once he was passing by a house when he saw a woman grinding jowar. He was moved to tears by the tragic fate of those seeds. He cried deeply like a child.They actually conveyed the impending death of man in a similar way. A sadhu who was passing by asked him for the reason of his sorrow and Kabir explained him the reason. The sadhu felt very much touched by his vairagya and explained him the philosophy of life from the very same example, "Look my son, the jowar seeds indeed explain the temporary life of man. But look carefully!!Few seeds stuck to the rod are intact.They cannot be crushed. In the same way a man who is stuck to the rod of God through bhakthi, though he is being grinded in the samsara will not be affected by death". Kabir was very much impressed by these words and dedicated his entire life in the path of bhakthi to God. What a great story indeed!! In one of his writings Kabir proclaims,

"moko kahan dhunde re baande?mein tho tere paas mein.
Na teerath mein na morath mein Naekanth nivas mein
Na mandir mein na masjid mein Na kashi kailash mein
Na japa mein na tapa mein Na mein vrat upas mein
Moko kahan dhunde re baande? Mein tho tere paas mein".

With these beautiful lines Kabir says God is with us and one should see God in everyone and everything in us.Only then one can see the true path of mukthi or liberation.

THE KEY TO JNANA

When we go into the hierarchy of our yoga, they say jnana yoga is superior than karma yoga.Maybe in the philosophical view and scripture view it's true. But according to many of our saints and myself I strongly believe

karma yoga is always at first place when it comes to practice.Anyways when coming to the path of jnana,we say, whenever a person gets detached from his karma he attains the path of jnana according to our ancient texts. Now you would probably ask me how is it in a normal living individual's life?It all begins with self introspection. Probably the best way of practicing jnana yoga is self introspection. Many of us have actually misunderstood jnana yoga as what we are getting through formal education. But jnana yoga is way beyond that. It comes only when you self introspect everyday and your entire karma and it's purpose for which the karma was based upon.Then slowly you start getting detached from your day to day actions. I am not saying you won't do work but your expectations associated with your action reduces. Then you would just have the willingness to work. Nomatter whether it benefits oneself or for the society, the person starts working with the same enthusiasm. The best words given by Shankaracharya was "Aham brahmasmi". The entire source of creation lies within me. But the maya which veils this aspect should be removed by continous introspection towards oneself. Why this birth? What is the purpose of my life? What is this birth and death cycle? Every creature on this earth has a purpose for which it is made. Probably all the creatures are fullling their purposes except man. The so called "intelligent creatures" are just going on with useless stuffs in day to day life instead of understanding the beautiful nature in and around them as Swami Vivekanada says," God manifested himself in the form of living creatures".This beautiful God picture lies surely in the eyes of the beholder.Yoga is one of the best tool in opening these eyes to see the God within us.

THE STORY OF JNANA

Once Shankaracharya was walking through the market place with his disciples. There he saw a man dragging a cow by a rope. Shankaracharya then told the man to wait and then asked his disciples to surround them. "I am going to teach you something", and then continued.... "Tell me who is bound to whom? Is the cow bound to this man or the man bound to this cow?" The disciples without hesitation said that the cow was bound to the man."The cow is bound to the man.The man is the master. He is holding the rope. The cow has to go wherever the master goes", said the disciples. "Now watch this", he then immediately took a scissor from his bag and cut the rope. The cow ran away from the master and the master ran after his cow. "Look, what is happening", said Shankaracharya, "Do you see who the Master is? The cow is not at all interested in this man. The cow in fact, is trying to escape from this man." This is the case with our MIND. Like the cow, all the non-sense that we carry inside is not interested in us. WE ARE INTERESTED IN IT, we are keeping it together somehow or the other. We are going crazy trying to keep it all together under our control. What a nice story indeed. Shankaracharya said to be the original propounder of jnana yoga through his advaitha vedantha teachings gave a base for the philosophy and practice of jnana yoga. According to him the two essential qualities of a seeker of jnana should be complete renunciation and deep desire for absolute liberation from maya or illusion. Yoga is one such self discipline practices that helps in estabilishing the non-dual experience of this formless divinity or in shankaracharya words called"advaitha jnana". It helps in winning over the "dvandvas" of our day to day life activities as patanjali says, "Tatho dvandva anabhigataha" leading to "samattva" or "balanced state of mind" which would surely stop the fights going on within our mind and help us unleashing the true knowledge or I would say the truth residing within us!!

FROM THE CONCENTRATION CAMPS

From my childhood I had these passionate thoughts about creation and it's purpose. What are we made for?There is a reason for everything in this planet.Then what could be the purpose All these reasons used to ponder me as a child growing up. We have certain pattern of life which we seem to follow knowingly or unknowingly.You might have seen small children learning to walk or speaking some things which wonders everyone. Who taught them all these? Then there should be some inner energy within us which is making all these stuffs.Exactly we cannot say as God because there are instances or greater minds who had doubts about god's existence.One should know that Stephen Hawking never believed that there was a creator of universe. Because according to him time never existed before creation. We cannot call his words as false because his

writings were exactly based on facts of time travel and there may be truth. But anyways more important aspect for us to think of, is the purpose for which we all have been made!! We all have been in the form of an abstract painting. It has a lot of meaning embedded within it but it's very hard to understand when just looked with a layman eyes. Only a good guy with good vision can appreciate it. Now moving on I had an eye opener in understanding about these aspects when I came across of the writings of great psychiatrist and also a neurologist Victor frankl.His experience in the concentration camps laid out by nazis whose leader as we all know was Adolf hitler. Being personally a survivor of this Holocaust, Victor frankl has explained the life one

had to undergo in these camps. This experience gave him an experience of what life actually is all about.The thing that matters the most is during all his struggle he found out the truth what yoga has also been focussing upon.We would move on with this experience of him in our next chapter!!

LIFE IN CONCENTRATION CAMPS

Now moving on you all probably would have heard about adolf hitler and his antisemitism. The life what the Jews underwent in the concentration camps due to the hatredness resulting in the death of 6 million Jews in the holocaust.This prejudice against the Jews were not just physical but this anitisemitism was more rather mental. For which even adolf hitler says he wanted it to be like that and it was even felt by all these prisoners.Whatever it is we have a lot to learn from these life experiences. One such experiences was from Victor frankl who was the survivor of this holocaust. In his writings he states the transition of emotions they underwent. Being himself a psychologist these experiences taught him what life actually is all about as he states. In these concentration camps people used to lose everything their possessions, wealth, goals everything and what alone remained was the last to freedom, the ability to choose one's attitude in a given set of circumstances. Though they were beaten with whips even for small and pesky reasons more than all these physical suerings it was the mental pain which seemed to be the worst!! At rst there was a curiosity that resulted for them imagining their plight, but later what turned out to be was apathy.They had to stand cleaning the railway tracks even amid bitter cold for almost hours and if anyone found to get little weakened or tired, the reward one would get would be from a whip. And suddenly one would start working again. One more worst was aroused along with these miseries which was nothing but typhus fever. This resulted in massive slaves to get turned into sick. Some of them were taken into sick rooms by a convoy. If found unable to recover they were sent to the gas chambers. Many of the prisoners who were also disobeying the orders of the capos and the SS men were also sent to these gas chambers where they were slaughtered to death.In all these concentration camps one could barely wish for was a piece of bread and watery soup. Even this was not provided adequately.They were just given these twice a day.Many times whenever there was a shift from concentration camps even this wouldn't be available.Sometimes they had to work over fields and many times people would be suffering from edema in their feet due to frostbite. But they tried to walk as properly as they can. Anyone found limping or weak were again would and themselves with more worst treatment by the capos. They were also shifted to sick camps making that as their last part of their life.Even in their dreams one would think of food.And one went on losing all these feelings towards others and the aspect of cynicism started to arouse later. Maybe it was the only way for their survival even though there was an instance of cannibalism seen.Even admist all of these situations there was a dream of

their previous life which made them move on further. The basic

instances of their life like closing a door, favourite food all these

thoughts were reminded to them even in these terrible situations. There was a transition from the state of

curiosity about
their plight to the state of apathy because of this continous suering. Many a times they would get horror dreams in sleep
but no one used to wake them up as what more worst could be
there than their present living life.Frankl in these all experiences says that life is not about pleasure as what freud proposed
or about power as said by psychologist adler but life is all about
a meaning.The understanding of existence of this meaning was
what led them to go through this fricken part of life successfully. Whenever the crowded train passed from one camp to another camp from auschwitz to bavaria through salzburg mountains all would rush to peep through the hole to see the mountains and the natural beauty with that small hole of light coming from outside. This was the beauty of life which made him
understand that life purely lies in the concept of existentialism.
or about power as said by psychologist adler but life is all about
a meaning.The understanding of existence of this meaning was
what led them to go through this fricken part of life successfully. Whenever the crowded train passed from one camp to another camp from auschwitz to bavaria through salzburg mountains all would rush to peep through the hole to see the mountains and the natural beauty with that small hole of light coming from outside. This was the

beauty of life which made him
understand that life purely lies in the concept of existentialism.

YOGA AND EXISTENTIALISM

When you are in an irrational universe you will actually make
rational decisions and try to and the beauty and purpose of life.

Coming all the way through the story of Viktor E frankl one could acknowledge that life bears something more of hidden meaning than just destiny and goals.What would it be? What made this great neurologist and psychiatrist to live for more than 3 years in that dreadful suffering?Had it not been he could have found relief by suicide or something more. But it was not the thing which he wished for. It was just his will for hope to live which made him bear all his suffering. This is what the principle of existentialism propounds in logotherapy as
third Viennese school of psychotherapy. Victor who was very much influenced by freud at first, later discovered that life was not just mere pleasure as Freud says or just the quest for power as adler, it was more than that. It was the will for meaning, in other words to go in search for the purpose of life. This purpose is not goals as we have in this materialistic world. It's something more to portrait at. It's the potential meaning hidden under each individual which

is unique in every individual as we have suffering to be unique in every individual.Many people in society keep on saying repeatedly that life is vague and they are helpless about it. But in real sense it's false. As Jean Paul Sartre, the founder of existentialism says, "Existence always preceedes the essence".The ability to choose our attitude under a given set of circumstances is what life is all about. Now this attitude and kind of suffering or enjoyment one undergoes is different in each individual.The kind of attitude we chose decides whether one "suffers in the suffering" Or "one comes out of this suffering". In today's world many people all over the world are seen to accept this concept of existentialism as it helps to overcome their boredom of life or in other words known as " Existential nullness".Unlike Freud or Adler's psychology concepts, Jean Paul sartre's existentialism has always something to deal with physical dimension of an individual. Now how existentialism is related to yoga would be your question? I was not at all aware about this existentialism so much until when I came across an IIT Guwahati journal which had a comparative study of sankhya yoga and existentialism.Going through this comparative study made me analyse how even sankhya yoga could relate to existentialism which our ancestors have spoken way back. Let me explain you about this in a simple way. Sankhya yoga always speaks about the reality concept and understanding reality as the only means of attaining salvation. Even in the Sartre existentialism the same truth is being spoken about and thus proving the similarities in eastern and western philosophies. The term "existence precedes essence"in existentialism speaks about the same aspect,understanding the reality of your existence can only lead to the nectar of truth i.e., salvation in terms of yoga. When you start realising this you have no reason to hate any situation or person in particular. Because you wish to find out a solution or an attitude to frame at every situation. Going on with a simple explanation which I had come across, we all would have been knowing there would be two idols in a temple. One made of bronze known as uthsava murthi and the other which is established stone idol, prathishtapitha murthi by means of pranaprathishta.I was not at all aware of why we actually have two murthis in a temple of the same God. Every ritual or the things our ancestors have done has some philosophical or scientic understanding to represent at!! As a child, seeing all the religious procession I used to feel that may be the stone idol is fixed and cannot be carried so they have made another one.Maybe you all would have thought the same thing probably.Now the bronze idol whatever we see is nothing but the individual self, it is just the representation of the soul or the stone idol or murthi of the temple. We all are carried away by this individual self like the bronze idol which looks beautiful with lights and decorations but the true permanent self resides in the prathishtapana murthi.Hence even when we oer something to the bronze idol it should always be directed to or in the name of the stone idol in the temple.The individual self which is carried by ego but the true soul is always pure and without ego. By this one example of Indian tradition we can say that God existed in the form of stone idol who later defines himself in the form of bronze idol. He has just taken a dierent form in the form of bronze idol. His essence may be in the bronze idol but his existence is always permanent in the stone idol. Sartrean existentialism and yoga both aim at freedom from suering. While existentialism speaks about to find a meaning in suering, yoga speaks about the reality of suering or dukha. Yoga propounds that there can be no pleasure without pain or suering and no pain or suering without pleasure. It always succeedes one after the other being the cause of each other successively. While yoga speaks to understand this reality by practice leading to experience and a particular attitude. Sartrean existentialism says experience will lead you to a particular practice by framing an attitude followed by one's decision.But both of their path have the same ending. To understand the cause of suering and feeling the suering and pleasure as same i.e.to nd a meaning in suering. When there is a meaning in life there should also be a meaning in suering. To live is to suer and to strive is to nd a meaning in suering as Dr Victor frankl says in existentialism.

When we understand this we all will start loving one another and the world or the universality of the world as yoga says!! "Salvation is only through love and in love", as Dr. Victor frankl says.This is the only way that makes us to get out from the fear of death and accept it as a form of our existence. Yes it do exists as a part of my life and I should accept it. But before that I must fulll something or the purpose or meaning what life has asked for.It is not we expecting something from the life but what we have gifted for this life which is expecting from us.If we understand this simple concept probably even the greatest suering what we call as death would surely nd a meaning.Hence Yoga is the one tool which could probably help you in understanding this purpose of your existence and meaning of life.Recently I was coming across this fact that the stone idol whatever we have seen speaks about the universality,or the truth.It is the true soul. It cannot be changed as the stone idol which has been established.We can only give them oerings like owers to stone. The oerings to the soul is not owers or anything as such but our actions or our attitude we choose under a defined set of circumstances.

THE ORIGIN OF YOGA

Now moving on to the practical part, let's know how yoga has originated. There are a lot of myths about the origin of yoga. I mean probably healthy philosophical thoughts too. Because yoga has been seen and propounded in every religious texts. Whether philosophy or practice, everywhere we can see the highlights of yoga. Let's consider the holy Bhagavadgita, it speaks about Raja yoga.Then many philosophers or

saints argue that yoga originates from Sri krishna himself. Then in another context we see Shiva being referred as Adiyogi. Yes of course the way he sits in dhyana and many of the yogis consider Shiva himself the origin for yoga. It is said that Shiva or the Adiyogi on the banks of Kantisarovar in the Himalayas propounded this knowledge of yogic science to the saptarishis making the way for origin of yoga.Same period Mahavir and

Buddha propounded their teachings whose extracts are also found in Yoga.Hence Yoga origin is never solely dedicated to a single person or a community. It has been the practice of God's who wanted to teach a better way of life propounded them through his messengers who may be the preachers we find in our ancient texts or the ancient famous saints or any religious gurus. Now before moving on further, let us understand how the

postures of Shiva and Vishnu both can be the origin of

Yoga themselves.Coming to Vishnu, the protector of the world he is always seen resting on the sheshnag in the form of yoga nidra. They say the entire cosmic consciousness resides within him. That is why we see the whole universe in krishna's avatar of Vishnu when he asks him to open his mouth.He is always seen closing his eyes and being in his cosmic universal consciousness. The day he opens his eyes, it means he is set out to eradicate the evil which has crossed the limit. Now coming to Lord shiva, though he is called as the destroyer he is a shantaswaroopi. He is

always seen meditating without any attachments. He takes on the burden of the world but with detachment.He is never connected to anyone.His posture always signifies the state of samadhi or the ultimate awareness towards himself.The Ganga river which flows from his head represents the immortal stream

of higher yogic consciousness.Now you might ask me How does he control the world without connecting? That is Shiva. He does that by focussing on the cosmic consciousness within himself with complete detachment of the world.He is often referred to as 'Tamasi'.Though we consider Shiva as being sattvic, being calm and simple always but when he is on the verge of destruction he has the Tamoguna, The character of ignorance where in this destructive mode he is referred as Rudra. Shiva has been said to be having four expansions namely Vasudeva, Pradyumna, Aniruddha and Sankarshana.Lord Shiva knows that Sankarsana is the original cause of his own existence, and thus he always meditates upon Him in trance. Because destruction is

in the mode of ignorance, Lord Shiva and his worshipable

Deity, Sankarsana, are technically called tamasi. Since both Lord Shiva and Sankarsana are always enlightened and situated in the transcendental position, they have nothing to do with the modes of material nature–goodness, passion and ignorance–but because

their activities involve them with the mode of ignorance, they are sometimes called tamasi. Shiva when he is calm and in yogic pose is referred as Dakshina moorthi.When we actually go into further deeper view it has been said that the adishesha always meditates or worships Shiva to actually view the tandav of him

in Vishnu's heart. Its also known as "Ajapa tandava" which makes Vishnu heavier due to the happiness within his heart.That's what you tend to feel in the ultimate state of yoga nidra whereas in the state of Shiva, he is in the calm state of samadhi of calmness whose restless energy are drawn upon by shakthi to make him control the world even in the detached state.So with all these stories around let's move on with the further practice

of yoga!!

THE PRACTICE OF YOGA

Now coming basically into the concept, how yoga should bepracticed?There are a lot of people who have different opinions regarding their practice. Some may prefer Hatha yoga or some may prefer Ashtanga yoga and so on. But what I believe in is that it always depends upon an individual and the way he has been composed which matters. It can always be known only by the person himself. Whatever that comes through the yoga gurus or the practitioners is just the light for the path of yogic discovery of oneself.But the complete knowledge about one's physical and mental status can only be known by the person himself.In a simple way if I can explain
this is by the concept of pain. Let's assume a patient approaches a doctor with some pain in some part of the body. The doctor can only get some part of information from his diagnosis. But majority of the information about his pain can only be got from the patients words or how he responds.So by understanding our
condition and our preferences we should go up with the practice, as there is no one who knows better about us than we ourselves. Whatever the form of yoga you believe in, I suggest to never jump into the yogic pose directly. It's always a wrong thing that people believe that yoga is just asanas whatever the form it is!! This should be overcome as yoga is just more than that.Each form of yoga has

something to speak about along with its practice. It's always necessary to understand those things which is necessary for gaining perks of our practice.Moving forward in the next chapters let's go on understanding about different forms of yoga and it's practice!!

A NOTE ON PATANJALI YOGA

This form of Yoga has been also referred to as Ashtanga yoga. It just not only involves the physical practice
but preceeding it one has to undergo a lot of preparations before actually going into the physical practice. These preparations can be more precisely some form of modifications in our mind as well as our qualities.I would rather say in yoga these qualities are described as yamas and niyamas.In ashtanga yoga
as I have felt these yamas and niyamas majorly act as gates in opening up the path for becoming yogi. More probably in our society as I have seen there has been a lot of confusions or misconceptions with regards to ashtanga yoga and vinyasa. Vinyasa is just a style of physical practice that has been developed and
evolved from Ashtanga yoga.But the Ashtanga yoga itself is entirely very much vast than vinyasa style. Now coming to theconcept of Ashtanga Yoga it involves eight limbs which form a firm foundation for it and hence derive its name as such.The eight limbs are

1. Yama
2. Niyama
3. Asana
4. Pranayama
5. Pratyahara
6. Dharana

7. Dhyana
8. Samadhi

Probably in all the traditional yoga books of Ashtanga yoga you can come across these eight limbs.These eight limbs are the ones which makes it emerge as popular across the globe.It not only aims at bringing out physical transformation alone but more precisely aims for spiritual transformation when compared with Hatha yoga which actually emphasizes on purification of body as well as nadis or energy channels. Now let us
move onto the very first limb Yama. It's further has been classified as 1)Ahimsa 2)Satya 3)Asteya 4)Brahmacharya 5)Aparigraha. Coming to the yamas, they are the ones which help oneself "to control".More precisely they help to tame the mind.Now coming to the first yama i.e., Ahimsa is rightly said as Non-violence. Though it just seems as a simple thing but practising it is one of the most difficult thing in today's society.
As we are all in a rat race, one going over the other for his needs, it's obvious that violence will occur.Basically one should always understand "Himsa" Or the "Violence" what here is referred to as is not just mere physical fights, but more than that!!
Violence can occur by Action, Words and our inner feelings towards the other, what we actually refer in sanskrit as Kaya,Vacha and Manasa. There are moments wherein I personally started practising Ahimsa but fact was that it seemed to be so much difficult. The first thing which seems to be physical is way more easier. Avoiding physical fights, but the latter ones increases the level of difficulty in practice as sometimes they never arise from

our conscious level. So the best thing what I would advice is staying calm.In many instances most of our problems gets sorted out just by staying calm.And also we must start praying to God and follow the path of Bhakthi yoga to refrain ourselves from the act of 'himsa'. We all should remember the Emperor Ashoka who gave away most of all his wealth in order to estabilish the message of "Peace" in India.Mind can be a friend to us as well as an enemy. Hence we must know the right path. Only the right thoughts bring in the right words and right words can bring in the right actions. This is how it works in a cycle.

Now coming to the second yama that is "Satya".Basically it's not just speaking truth to everyone. It's actually being truthful to oneself. We make so many promises in day to day lives particularly with our ownselves. I would do that thing, I would do this work and so on. But as the time progresses we just postpone it and forget the promises which we have made to ourselves. So at first we must all start being truthful to oneself before actually being truthful towards others, as they say what comes from within stays outside. Next we will move on to Asteya or Non Stealing.Its always said to estabilish "Sarva ratna" according to the sutras of patanjali in the sadhana pada.Asteya is not just mere non stealing of physical objects but it has way far concept than this. We should never try to obstruct other's ideas and desires.We should have an awareness of what belongs to us and

what doesn't, be it physical objects or ideas or desires. One must understand that when the heart is pure everything comes to us as explained in the laws of karma.

Next let's move on to Brahmacharya or what we term as celibacy.As a quote goes "Truth is what we are".Now how

to discover it? It can be only done by Brahmacharya.Brahmacharya when split it two words we get
the terms "Brahma" meaning "Infinity" and "charya" means "moving".So moving towards the infinity within you always represents the brahmacharya. Its not just about not marrying someone but it's like being able to practice the brahmacharya yoga where we start getting awareness that we are not just body but more beyond that.When we start experiencing this infiniteness we actually start feeling joyful. And when we start feeling joyful,
the lighter the body becomes. We tend to go towards tha subtle aspect within us and we actually go beyond our senses. When this brahmacharya is established, we derive the infinite source of energy within us what is termed as "veeryalabaha". Next moving on to the last yama known as " Aparigraha" or Non-accumulation. Be it whatever, we should always try to subside the greed which is present within us. The need to accumulate more and more should always be cut down. As a proverb goes "When you give, you gain more. Whatever you scatter you have it all. What you hold on to,You lose that also".Explaining it in a simple way you know how to earn grain for food.You will earn for it but in the same way what happens if out of greed we start accumulating more and more of it in a store room, it gets spoiled.

Same thing happens even with all the other aspects if man is filled with the excess desire within himself.

Next let's move on to the Niyamas or what is termed as rules or regulations. They are as follows: 1)Shaucha 2)Santosha 3)Tapas 4)Swadhyaya 5)Ishwarapranidhana

Shaucha has been termed as "Cleanliness" Or more

precisely can be said as "purity".Not just purity of body but of mind,speech and action.As Sarada devi says " Pure mind always begets ecstatic love or prema bhakthi."When this purity develops, it helps in purification and experiencing the sattva within you. Next

moving to the Santosha or happiness. Saucha and santosha always go hand in hand. If there is no purity in any level there is no joy or happiness.A man becomes victim of disease either physical or mental and gets devoided from experiencing the happiness.And santosha is not just happiness it's also can be said as contentment. Feeling happy with what one has. If one starts feeling happy, all his desires gets subdued and

there is no chance of origin of miseries in his life.Hence one needs to be happy and contended with what one has and experience the real meaning of life. Tapas or austerity is termed as discipline in one's way of living. The word Tapas is derived from the word "tap" Which means "to burn". Tapas can mean cultivating a sense of self-discipline, passion and courage in order to burn away 'impurities' physically, mentally and emotionally,

and paving the way to our true greatness. Swadhyaya or " Self study is the next niyama which speaks on that one must always develop the habit or hunger for seeking more and more knowledge. This can be succeeded only when starts doing self study.Its not only just the study of scriptures or books but it is also the study of self as what lies within oneself.

Moving on with the last niyama that is Ishwarapranidhana.Fixing oneself towards the ultimate purusha who is also known as paramaguru that is Ishwara. Ishwara is more beyond than a personal God to anyone.

He is a spiritual significance for those who are in a yogic path to achieve emancipation or freedom from the attachments of worldly objects.

A NOTE ON PATHANJALI YOGA

The last three limbs of Ashtanga yoga — dharana, dhyana(meditation) and samadhi (enlightenment) — are collectively referred to as samyama, which means "control."

Next limb of patanjali yoga after pratyahara is "Dharana".Its been termed as "Concentration" Or "One pointed awareness".

When a man withdraws his senses, he has to focus his awareness or concentration to any point or object which can be external like any symbol or object or it can be internal as such by focussing on the chakras of our body.But for achieving Dharana one must be completely attained the perfect stages of pratyahara

or withdrawal of senses. After having one pointed awareness or focus forming the basis it leads to the next stage or limb of Patanjali yoga known as "Dhyana".Its been described as allowing our consciousness to flow in an uninterrupted way.This consciousness may be felt on physical level as creative ideas which tend to bring about a sense of bliss at the ultimate level. One starts to move on from a physical level to the metaphysical level. He moves on from the conscious to the subconscious state of mind unveiling his true self. This leads to the last stage or limb of the patanjali yoga what is known as "Samadhi".It can be achieved only when the sadhaka is absorbed in the object or objective of his meditation devoid of any other thoughts. If in that meditative state, only the object is present, without any modification of mind, that is samadhi.Here in this ultimate state the consciouness of the object shines whereas the consciousness of the self(svarupa) becomes empty. Samadhi is the gift that the yogi receives through the grace of God (ātmā). With samādhi the yogi has reached the goal, yoga as a method has led him to yoga as a conscious state of unity.

A NOTE ON HATHA YOGA -1

After speaking so much about patanjali yoga it would be unfair if we just miss out another important form of yoga which is Hatha yoga.I exactly still don't know whether it's easy or difficult to practise as there are still discussion among people between patanjali yoga and hatha yoga to know which suits best for a beginner.There has been no proper answer for this as both have their own principles which still makes anyone to get confused as which should be accepted. Hatha yoga always stresses upon shatkarmas to be practised before the actual practise of yama, niyama, asana and pranayama whereas patanjali yoga goes in a reverse order and says that mind should be tamed first by the practise of yamas and niyamas.Basically I personally suggest any beginner could actually start practising Hatha yoga as it doesn't involve so much vigorous flow as seen in Ashtanga or Patanjali yoga. After few stages of practice of Hatha yoga if he wishes he could then shift to Patanjali yoga. The word 'Ha' means Sun, 'tha' means Moon. Hatha means to balance the Sun and Moon energies in you. Hatha yoga is the science of harmonizing Pingala and Ida; or the solar and lunar energies within us so as to reach our higher consciousness to life. It is the science of activating the third, central nadi- Sushumna - which is the path to enlightenment. It is the

form which is most popular among the yogis of the Natha tradition. Patanjali yoga may accept other gods but Hatha yogis always accept or believe in
the Adinatha. In sanskrit "natha" means "Lord, protector" and Adinatha refers to the "first Lord" Or more precisely the "Original God".Basically these people of Nath cult are followers of extreme shaivism. Hence they always worship Lord shiva and believe he is the origin for Yoga. According to Hindu legends, Lord Shiva is credited with propounding Hatha yoga.It is said that on a lonely island,assuming nobody else would hear him,
he gave this knowledge of Hatha yoga to his wife Goddess Parvathi-but a fish heard the entire discourse, remaining still throughout.The fish later became a siddha which was transformed by Shiva himself out of kindness. He came to be known as Matsyendranath.Matsyendranath taught hatha yoga to his disciple Gorakshanath and to a limbless man, Chaurangi. Hatha yoga was thus passed down in disciplinic succession. Historically, classical Hatha Yoga is described primarily in three texts of Hinduism: Hatha Yoga Pradipika by yogi Swatmarama (15th centrury BCE), Shiva Samhita by unnkown author (~16th centrury BCE) and Gheranda Samhita by yogi Gheranda (17th century BCE). The major text Hatha yoga pradipika written by
Swatmarama is based on four aspect in introducing system, which is based on asanas (physical postures) and pranayama(breathing techniques) as a preparatory stage for physical purification of the body for the purpose of higher meditation or Yoga. Hatha Yoga Pradipika includes information about shatkarma (purication), chakras (centers of energy) and nadis (energy channels), kundalini (instict or female energy coiled at the

base of spine), bandhas (muscular locks), kriyas (cleansing techniques), Shakti (sacred force) and mudras (symbolic gestures) among other topics.Lets move on with all these aspects in my next chapter!!

A NOTE ON HATHA YOGA -2

Let's discuss about the views of Hatha yoga from one of the major texts i.e.Hatha yoga pradipika. The word "pradipika" means "to shed light" and Hatha yoga Pradipika hence acts as a guide in unvieling the dark mystery of Hatha yoga. Hatha yoga has been always described as a path one takes to reach the Raja yoga or previously discussed patanjali yoga. Basically the Hatha yoga Pradipika is divided

into four parts, The first explains yamas(control over behaviour), niyamas(rules and regulations), asanas(posture) and food.

The second one explains about pranayamas(control of energy) and shatkarmas(internal control of energy). The third deals with the mudras(seals), bandhas(lock), nadis(channels of energy through which prana flows) and the kundalini power. The fourth expounds pratyahara(withdrawal of senses),dharana(concentration),dhyana(meditation) and samadhi(absorption).

Now let me go on explaining about some new aspects which are different and more stressed in Hatha yoga rather than our repeated discussion of same things explained in patanjali yoga because I feel I have explained most of the topics in patanjali yoga itself. Now in the first part of Hatha yoga more stress is also given on diet along with asanas, yamas and niyamas.Many a times I have wondered and loved the way they have explained diet in Hatha yoga. Anyone who actually comes across diet part in Hatha yoga would actually start following it if he gets to know about it properly. The food according to Hatha yoga has been divided into three:

1)Sattvic 2)Tamasic 3)Rajasic

Sattvic food: This type of food is very good for mind.This type of food makes one's mind steady and avoids

the fluctuations.More than all of these I have personally experienced the lightness in one's own body when he actually goes for it. Sattvic food increases the duration of life and increases the purity of one's own bodily existence.It gives strength, stamina, health and happiness. The food coming under sattvic category are green vegetables, milk and milk products, seeds, sprouted seeds, honey, legumes, fruit, fruit juices, etc,… Hatha yoga always recommends one to take sattvic food to keep healthy body and mind.Foods like mung beans, wheat,rice shashtika,barley, milk, ghee, sugar,.etc, can be taken.The yogi should take nourishing and sweet food mixed with ghee and milk; it should nourish the dhathus (basic body constituents) and be pleasing

and suitable.

Tamasic food:If sattvic food represents purity, tamasic food

represents inertia, dullness or a state of inactivity.It may be good while having it sometimes but later it leads to dullness. It leads to a state of ignorance.The foods coming under this category are meat, alcohol, tobacco, Fermented food.

Rajasic food:Rajasic food stimualates the mind. It is known

to hyperexcite the nervous system in man. Even though it may feel good while eating, it actually causes the disturbance in mind-body equilibrium. The foods coming under this category are very hot, spicy, sour, salty or dry foods, tea, coffee, onion, garlic, eggs are coming under this category.Eating in hurried is also considered as Rajasic.

Now knowing about all these, what should be the quantity or amount of food one should consume?

Hatha yoga even explains the same concept as Mitahara in the following manner :

Susnigdha madhurahara chaturthamshavivarjitaha Bhujyate shiva samprityi mitaharaha sa uchyate'

Mitahara is always said to be agreeable and sweet food, leaving one-fourth of the stomach free and eaten(as an offering to Lord shiva). This clearly says that one should not over eat at all, Half of the stomach should be filled with solid food, remaining one fourth one has to take water, and one should keep last one fourth free. The beauty of this is it explains that whatever the food we consume should always be felt as an offering to Lord shiva who resides within us, making us to leave our egoistic and "I"ness attitude to subdue within us. Coming to asanas, of all the Asanas, Siddhasana, Padmasana, Simhasana,and Bhadrasana, are the very highest. They should always be practiced as a process of purification and to free oneself from fatigue more than

just physical exercise according to Hatha yoga. Next let's move on with the Shatkarmas Pranayama, Kumbhaka,Bandhas and Mudras in our next chapter!!

A NOTE ON HATHA YOGA -3

Now let's move on with our discussion with on Mudras discussed in Hatha yoga. The mudras that have been mentioned basically in Hatha yoga are as follows:

1. Mahamudra
2. Mahabandha mudra
3. Mahavedha mudra
4. Kechari mudra
5. Vipareethakarini mudra
6. Vajroli mudra
7. Mahamudra:Having pressed the perineum with the heel of the left foot and stretched out the right leg one should firmly hold the toe.With the throat locked,one should restrain the prana where he bends his neck backward to look up and should assume the position of a coiled serpant , which has been struck

by a stick. Then, the curved and evasive Kundalini suddenly, becomes forcefully straight.After Kumbhaka one should breathe out slowly and softly. This is the Mahamudra whose regular practice reduces the bondage or afflictions(kleshas)and death is improved.

8. Mahabandha mudra:With the heel of the left foot press the perineum. Then place the right foot on the left thigh. Firmly press the chin on the chest and inhaling, focus the chitta on the middle Nadi. One should practice kumbhaka to one's capacity and then exhale.One should practice on

the right side after having practised on the left side This is Mahabandha mudra.

9. Mahavedha mudra:The fully concentrated Yogi seated in Mahabandha should inhale. With the throat mudra he should restrain the breath. Placing both palms on the side of the body he should slowly beat the buttocks against the ground. This causes the air to leave the other Nadis and flow through the middle nadi.The Moon nadi, the Sun nadi and the Fire nadi having been joined together bestow the nectar of immortality.

4)Kechari mudra:When the tongue in the reverse direction enters the skull cavity, Kechari mudra occurs. Those

who cannot reach the tongue to skull cavity can start practicing to touch the backside of the upper palate. The tongue in the reverse position be taken to a place where the three paths come together. It is called the "Vyoma Chakra".This is called as Kechari mudra.Kechari mudra has been found to be very much beneficial in most of the disorders and frees oneself from the effect of poison, disease, old age, yawning, sleep, thirst,swoon,hunger and death.

5)Vipareethakarini mudra:Lie on the back. The arms are straight, beside the body.Inhaling, bend the knees and raise the legs and buttocks. Bring the hands under the hips to support the buttocks. Elbows remain on the floor. Straighten the legs vertically upwards. Relax the muscles of the feet, legs and hips.

Breathing normally, remain in this position as long as comfortable. Exhale, bend the knees towards the forehead, slowly lower the buttocks and legs, and return to the starting position.

1. Vajroli mudra:Sahajoli and Amaroli are the two varieties of Vajroli mudra. The Yogi unmindful of any worldly behaviour, after mixing the two juices should smear his limbs with pure ashes soaked in water. Yoga even practices for pleasure bestows liberation.Here it requires the yogin to preserve his semen, either by learning not to release it, or if released by drawing it up through his urethra from the vagina of "a woman devoted to the
practice of yoga".It is not practised in recent times as it may result in legal issues sometimes. This practice has been proposed to serve to clean the bladder by drawing liquids towards the urethra as an auto-enema, similar to the intestinal shatkarma of basti. This was all about a brief discussion about Hatha yoga
concepts as well as it's practice.

A NOTE ON HATHA YOGA-4

After knowing about diet and asanas in Hatha yoga, let's move on with the next concept i.e., Shatkarmas or Shatkriyas. In sanskrit "Shat" means "six".Hence it involves six purification process for a healthy body and mind. They are as follows: 1)Dhauti 2)Basti 3)Neti 4)Trataka 5)Nauli 6)Kapalabhati

1. Dhauti kriya:Here the sadhaka, according to the directions of his Guru should slowly swallow a wet piece of cloth, which is four fingers wide. He should then pull out that piece of wet cloth. This is called Dhauti karma according to Hatha yoga. It is said to be very much beneficial in breathing difficulties and I have been said that it is very much good in skin conditions. Also I have seen the glow in one's face after the practice of this kriya.

2. Basti kriya:In a squatting position, in water upto the navel with a tube inserted into the anus and contracting the rectum so that water will be sucked inside, the washing of the organ of excretion is called Basti kriya.A bamboo tube six fingers long is called as Basti.Four fingers length of it is inserted into the rectum and two finger length should remain outside.Edema, Stomach ailments, Gas, excessive pitta.etc., will become well balanced by the practice of Basti kriya.

3. Neti kriya:Here the sadhaka pulls out of the mouth a soft string of the circumference of one hand after having

made it pass through the nostrils. The neti kriya helps in the purification of the brain and head, bestows divine vision on the sadhaka, and removes all diseases.

4.Trataka kriya:A well composed and completely attentive sadhaka, should steadily gaze, fix his eyes on a target until the tears are shed. This is known as Trataka according to hatha yoga text. This trataka is the healer

of eye diseases and the remover of drowsiness.

5)Nauli kriya:Bend the shoulders forward and rotate the abdominal muscles to the right and left quickly like a whirlpool.This practice is called Nauli kriya by the siddhas. It increases the fire in the belly and removes digestive disorders.It gives bliss for the Sadhaka and removes all disorders.

6)Kapalabhati kriya:The process of releasing and drawing in breath quickly like a bellows is well known as Kapalabhati.This Kriya is the well known remover of ailments of Kapha. There is one more kriya known as Gajakarani kriya. Here the sadhaka vomits the contents of the stomach after drawing the apana upto the throat.By the regular and routine practice of this technique the intestines are mastered. It is also referred to as "Elephant instrument". Hatha yoga always recommends the practice of shatkarmas before beginning with pranayama. The major thing explained in pranayama of hatha yoga is that it majorly stresses on breath retention or kumbhaka. It says that as long as the breath is retained in the body, so long as the Chitta is undisturbed,and so long as the gaze is fixed between the two eyebrows, there is no fear of death.

Pranayama is said to have consisting three techniques according to hatha yoga:

1)Pooraka(Inhaling)

2)Rechaka(Exhaling)
3)Kumbhaka(Retention)

As long as the Kevala Kumbhaka has not been accomplished, the duration of the Sahitha kumbhaka has to be practiced to extend it(pranayama with both internal and external breath retention).Kevala Kumbhaka is a state where inhalation and exhalation are not considered as necessary. It is in par with the samadhi state.The easy and comfortable suspension of the prana without releasing out or drawing in is called Kevala Kumbhaka. In later advanced stages of practice one could go with the practice of Bandhas and mudras.There are mainly three types of Bandhas namely:

4. Jalandhara Bandha
5. Uddiyana Bandha
6. Moola Bandha.

When all these three Bandhas are performed at the same time it's called as "Maha Bandha".

Let's move on with the practice of first Bandha i.e.Jalandhara Bandha. Jalandhara bandha is said to be the holder of water. It binds the network of nadis and prevents the downward flow of water. It is the destroyer of throat misery. It involves inhaling and bending your neck forward and contraction of the throat. It is found to be very much beneficial in thyroid disorders. Uddiyana bandha involves the contraction of the abdomen. Uddiyana means to fly. By the practise of uddiyana bandha, the bound prana flies up to the sushumna like a bird. Pull back the abdomen by all might with deep inhalation and raise it above the navel.This practice is called as Uddiyana bandha, like a lion to kill the elephant of death. It is said that even an old man who practices

uddiyana bandha as instructed by guru regains youth. Lastly comes the Moolabandha or the Anal lock. Here the Anus should be firmly contracted while pressing the perineum with the heel to pull up
the Apana.This lock making the normally down and out flowing Apana(one of the five subdivisons of prana and this energy is believed to flow downwards and outwards, influencing the digestion,elimination and reproduction)go upward is called as Mulabandha. Having pressed the door of the anus, the Sadhaka should
pull up the Apana repeatedly and forcefully so that it rises.

BEYOND THE "I"

After knowing about diet and asanas in Hatha yoga, let's move on with the next concept i.e., Shatkarmas or Shatkriyas. In sanskrit "Shat" means "six".Hence it involves six purification process for a healthy body and mind. They are as follows: 1)Dhauti 2)Basti 3)Neti 4)Trataka 5)Nauli 6)Kapalabhati

1. Dhauti kriya:Here the sadhaka, according to the directions of his Guru should slowly swallow a wet piece of cloth, which is four fingers wide. He should then pull out that piece of wet cloth. This is called Dhauti karma according to Hatha yoga. It is said to be very much beneficial in breathing difficulties and I have been said that it is very much good in skin conditions. Also I have seen the glow in one's face after the practice of this kriya.

2. Basti kriya:In a squatting position, in water upto the navel with a tube inserted into the anus and contracting the rectum so that water will be sucked inside, the washing of the organ of excretion is called Basti kriya.A bamboo tube six fingers long is called as Basti.Four fingers length of it is inserted into the rectum and two finger length should remain outside.Edema, Stomach ailments, Gas, excessive pitta.etc., will become well balanced by the practice of Basti kriya.

3. Neti kriya:Here the sadhaka pulls out of the mouth a soft string of the circumference of one hand after having

made it pass through the nostrils. The neti kriya helps in the purification of the brain and head, bestows divine vision on the sadhaka, and removes all diseases.

4.Trataka kriya:A well composed and completely attentive sadhaka, should steadily gaze, fix his eyes on a target until the tears are shed. This is known as Trataka according to hatha yoga text. This trataka is the healer

of eye diseases and the remover of drowsiness.

5)Nauli kriya:Bend the shoulders forward and rotate the abdominal muscles to the right and left quickly like a whirlpool.This practice is called Nauli kriya by the siddhas. It increases the fire in the belly and removes digestive disorders.It gives bliss for the Sadhaka and removes all disorders.

6)Kapalabhati kriya:The process of releasing and drawing in breath quickly like a bellows is well known as Kapalabhati.This Kriya is the well known remover of ailments of Kapha. There is one more kriya known as Gajakarani kriya. Here the sadhaka vomits the contents of the stomach after drawing the apana upto the throat.By the regular and routine practice of this technique the intestines are mastered. It is also referred to as "Elephant instrument". Hatha yoga always recommends the practice of shatkarmas before beginning with pranayama. The major thing explained in pranayama of hatha yoga is that it majorly stresses on breath retention or kumbhaka. It says that as long as the breath is retained in the body, so long as the Chitta is undisturbed,and so long as the gaze is fixed between the two eyebrows, there is no fear of death.

Pranayama is said to have consisting three techniques according to hatha yoga:

1)Pooraka(Inhaling)

2)Rechaka(Exhaling)

3)Kumbhaka(Retention)

As long as the Kevala Kumbhaka has not been accomplished, the duration of the Sahitha kumbhaka has to be practiced to extend it(pranayama with both internal and external breath retention).Kevala Kumbhaka is a state where inhalation and exhalation are not considered as necessary. It is in par with the samadhi state.The easy and comfortable suspension of the prana without releasing out or drawing in is called Kevala Kumbhaka. In later advanced stages of practice one could go with the practice of Bandhas and mudras.There are mainly three types of Bandhas namely:

4. Jalandhara Bandha
5. Uddiyana Bandha
6. Moola Bandha.

When all these three Bandhas are performed at the same time it's called as "Maha Bandha".

Let's move on with the practice of first Bandha i.e.Jalandhara Bandha. Jalandhara bandha is said to be the holder of water. It binds the network of nadis and prevents the downward flow of water. It is the destroyer of throat misery. It involves inhaling and bending your neck forward and contraction of the throat. It is found to be very much beneficial in thyroid disorders. Uddiyana bandha involves the contraction of the abdomen. Uddiyana means to fly. By the practise of uddiyana bandha, the bound prana flies up to the sushumna like a bird. Pull back the abdomen by all might with deep inhalation and raise it above the navel.This practice is called as Uddiyana bandha, like a lion to kill the elephant of death. It is said that even an old man who practices uddiyana bandha as instructed by guru regains youth. Lastly comes the Moolabandha or the Anal lock. Here the Anus should be firmly contracted while pressing the perineum with the heel to pull up

the Apana.This lock making the normally down and out flowing Apana(one of the five subdivisons of prana and this energy is believed to flow downwards and outwards, influencing the digestion,elimination and reproduction)go upward is called as Mulabandha. Having pressed the door of the anus, the Sadhaka should

pull up the Apana repeatedly and forcefully so that it rises.

PANCHAKOSHA CONCEPT OF YOGA IN THERAPY

As said earlier I am a great fanatic when it comes with understanding human psychology. It seems so much interesting for me to know how well our thoughts can be seen on any given aspect and how each individual views vary when shown with any object or concept. It never seems always the same. In fact particularly I have seen the arise of new thoughts or views about the same fact or object in discussion.It also gives me so much interest to know how we have been evolved psychologically. In this conquest I have come across western theories as well as our own Indian theories and one such Indian concept was our Panchakosha theory. Let's also understand how well this can be used psychologically in getting freedom from a variety of our illnesses. Recently I was coming across a journal article by Dr.Biswajit satpathy which spoke about the Panchakosha theory of personality which has been mentioned in Taittiriya upanishad. Now let's see some of its highlights. This is said to be the vedantic psychophilosophical view of human personality. According to this theory, human body consists of five sheaths:

1)"Annamaya kosha", a segment of body nourished by food.

2) "Pranamaya kosha", segment nourished by prana i.e.,

bioenergy.

3) "Manomaya kosha", segment nourished by education.

4) "Vijnanamaya kosha", segment nourished by ego.

5) " Anandamaya kosha", segment nourished by emotions.

These five koshas are said to be the five sheaths of human personality.Human body has three bodies where all these sheaths reside. They are:

1. Gross body(Sthula sharira)
2. Astral body(Linga sharira)
3. Causal body(Karana sharira)

Karana Sharira or Causal body is the map template which is the sole cause for the gross and subtle bodies. Pranamaya Kosha, movement of the pranic force directs our physical and mental activities. The Linga sharira(subtle body) surrounds the Sthula Sharira (physical body) as an aura of energy. A person who predominantly resides in Annamaya kosha believes that he is only the physical body and gives more importance to physical things. Such persons are good sports men and love physical fitness programs like games, sports, aerobics, Karate, body building, physical comfort, food, dress etc.,. A person who experiences Pranamaya kosha believe for a time that he is the inner energy animating the physical form and gives importance to pranayamas and meditation. Such people are very active and energetic. The person residing in the next kosha i.e., Manomaya kosha has thoughts and desires which identify with form and name, position and qualities. He is emotional in nature.This person lacks the cognitive ability of thinking and voids discrimination. But he may have very keen appreciation for fine arts, music,dance and drama. Next comes the person residing in Vijnanamaya kosha who is knowledgeable and wise,loves literature, creative and are good orators.The fourth sheath is the wisdom that lies beneath the processing, the thinking aspect of the mind.Person in this kosha is knowledgeable and wise.He loves literature, creative and are good orators. This fourth sheath is the wisdom that lies beneath the processing, thinking aspect of the mind.Discovery,research and management are the areas where these people are involved with. Next is the Anandamaya kosha which resides in the innermost sheath. Persons experiencing Anandamaya kosha are stable in behaviour and firm in decision,are happy in every state of life and they appreciate higher order of things and thinking like nature and connection with God etc., They are self realised persons. Now question arises is how this knowledge of koshas can be used as a therapy?The answer is simple, we have seen the qualities of a person in each kosha, so if anyone is disturbed, in any kosha there is outcome of disease. Like for example, if person has physical symptom, it may be from annamaya kosha. If he is having mental disorder, then disease may be from mind i.e.,manomaya kosha. Hence by knowing the cause, therapy can be administered to that kosha like by practising meditation if manomaya kosha is affected in a person. But one must be aware that a disease can penetrate into multiple koshas as well. Like for example,a person may be showing physical symptoms because of a disturbed mind also, like nosebleeds in hypertension.The symptoms is physical and one may think annamaya kosha but the more than that the causal and major kosha affected there is manomaya kosha. To know more exactly let's understand the path of disease with respect to the panchakosha theory. When we come to the Panchakosha concept,it says that the causes for disease is

due to kleshas or simply called as bondages.The purpose of yoga is to lessen the effect of these factors(klesha tanukaranam) and promote the state of integration(samadhi bhavanam). Now when it comes to these bondages, any normal person can understand that it arises from mind i.e., manomaya kosha. So manomaya kosha is the gateway for all the diseases. From here the disease progresses on to the vijnanamaya kosha. When the disease is present in these two koshas, the diseases is said to be in psychic phase.When disease progresses to the pranamaya kosha from vijnanamaya it is called psychosomatic phase.When this disease further progresses, one begins to identify the disease as there is damage to the target
specific organs. This phase is known as Somatic phase. If the disease manifests completely with pathological changes such as ulcerated stomach or chronic hypertension, manifesting in their totality resulting in complications.This phase can be correlated with the disease progressed to annamaya not only produces psychological and emotional distress but also leads to the termination of life of that person. Hence being a yoga practitioner or yoga therapist, one's prime duty is to find where the disease has been progressed and which kosha has been affected. This can be understood by seeing or experiencing some of the qualities which are very particular to each kosha. In this way one must try to understand Panchakosha as a personality or behaviour pattern of individuals and can be effectively used in yogic therapy.

YOGA AS A THERAPY

From my childhood days, I had these passionate thoughts about creation and it's purpose. What are we made for? There is a reason for everything in this planet.Then what could be the purpose of existence of we as humans on this planet? All these reasons used to ponder me as a child growing up. We have certain pattern of life which we seem to follow knowingly or unknowingly.You might have seen small children learning to walk or speaking some things which wonders everyone. Who taught them all these? Then there should be some inner energy within us which is making all these stuffs.Exactly we cannot say as God because there are instances or views by greater minds who had doubts about god's existence.One should know that Stephen Hawking never believed that there was a creator of universe. Because according to him time never existed before creation. We cannot call his words as false because his writings were exactly based on facts of time travel and there may be truth. But anyways more important aspect for us to think of, is the purpose for which we all have been made!! We all have been potrayed in the form of an abstract painting. It has a lot of meaning embedded within it but it's very hard to understand when just looked with a layman eyes. Only a good guy with good vision can appreciate it. Now moving on, I had an eye opener in understanding about these aspects when I came across with the writings of a great psychiatrist and also a neurologist Victor frankl.His experience in the concentration camps laid out by nazis whose leader as we all know was Adolf hitler. Being personally a survivor of this Holocaust, Victor frankl has explained the life one had to undergo in these camps. This experience gave him a view of what life actually is all about.The thing that matters the most is during all his struggle he found out the truth what yoga has also been focussing upon.We would move on with this experience of him in our next chapter!!

THE THEORY OF CAUSE AND EFFECT

Anyone who starts understanding cosmology will always begin with some of the concepts like the origin of Universe. Basically we all have been wondering about the evolution of the Universe. How all the stars came into being? How all the galaxies were formed ? How the solar system was formed? How planets came into being? How all of us have evolved ? Man is trying to find out answers to all of these questions and one answer that has been found out till now is the Big Bang theory. It says that all these galaxies, stars and planets ,every matter in the universe evolved from a single primordial ball of fire.This primordial ball burst out and resulted in the universe and the matter within it spread all along the entire universe. Now the question was who created that primordial ball with such enormous amount of matter and energy? Again people started propounding the existence of God and said that it was God who had placed that primordial ball of fire.The main reason for this was our concept of cause and effect!! We all have been believing from our childhood that for every effect there is a cause behind it. Of course it may be true in many of the aspects but it is always not true when it comes to the entire universe. Whether complex or subatomic, each and every matter behaves the same when viewed accurately. The best example is the protons at subatomic level which tend to originate from somewhere, collide and stick to each other,disappear and reappear again at some other point thus obeying the Laws of nature. The same thing is proposed by Stephen Hawking that even the primordial ball of universe containing all the entire universe would have evolved out as it was also made of same particles in the subatomic level. Hence there was a collision of this complex matter of primordial ball in the big bang resulting in the expansion of universe.But the answer to the question for the evolution of primordial ball is "nothing" which holds good even for the subatomic particles as said before which evolve and disappear from "nothing".Time never existed before creation and hence no one could have created the universe. It just could have been from the laws of nature.This theory completely opposes the existence of universe created by God by denying the theory of cause and effect as stated by Hawking. We even find the same discussion in Advaitha vedantha wherein they say God is beyond desires and to our perception of senses. If so, then why did he create the universe? Was it for his personal benefit or for some personal gratification? Then we all will agree that he cannot be the God In true sense and creator of course. He cannot be the moderator of cause and it's effects out there. According to us God should be beyond arishadvargas.Then when I was looking into this, I found one more nice thing which actually made me to arrive at one point. In philosophical point of view they say God created universe for "nothing". It was just a divine play, like children building a sand castle. There won't be any purpose as such. This is what we call as “Divine leela”. So when we put together all these we can always say our universe(primordial ball of fire in big bang)evolved from “Nothing”.And we should always accept that " The theory of Cause and effect never holds good for the entire world. As such with the creation of universe, it never holds good.Therefore in this world we can see so many effects without a cause like some diseases, sufferings and pains which do not have a cause as such but affect us when the whole world is taken into account.We see so much healthy people dying early without a a particular cause and hence it never holds good always. To understand and unleash the real mystery of this universe can be done only by looking scientifically in the universe by making use of science. Another way is looking deep within oneselves in search of the cosmic energies driven within us.Lets start discovering the beauty and truths about the cosmic universe situated above us and also deep within us through Science and Yoga respectively.

THE ESSENCE OF GITA

Bhagavad gita, is regarded as the holy book of Hindus. But more than all these its a message to the whole world irrespective of religion about how to be in one's life. All the holy scriptures of every religion teach us the same message. Love and compassion towards each other and surrenderance to the ultimate reality of nature. Now let's see about the Bhagavad gita. This epic poem has given a lot of answers to many of the people's questions and on the contrary raised a few questions also I suppose. The gita is a message by the Lord to the whole world mainly to those who seek refuge in him. For those who haven't had the pleasure of reading it, the Gita recounts a dialogue between Arjuna, one of five Pandava princes, and the Hindu deity Krishna, who in this epic serves as Arjuna's charioteer. Arjuna and his brothers have been exiled from the kingdom of Kurukshetra for 13 years and cut off from their rightful heritage by another faction of the family; the Gita takes up their struggle to reclaim the throne, which requires that Arjuna wage war against his own kinsmen, bringing his considerable military skills to bear.

The story begins on the dusty plains of Kurukshetra, where
Arjuna, a famed archer, is poised to fight. But he hesitates.He
sees arrayed against him friends, teachers, and kin, and believes
that to fight—and likely kill—these men would be to commit
a grievous sin and could bring nothing good even if he were to
win the kingdom back. Krishna chides him for his cowardice
—Arjuna is from the warrior caste after all, and warriors are meant to fight—but then goes on to present a spiritual rationale
for battling his enemies, one that encompasses a discussion of
the karma, jnana and bhakti yogas, as well as the nature of divinity, humankind's ultimate destiny, and the purpose of mortal
life. Now the real fact is not about this battle and krishna's upadesha.Have we ever wondered how Krishna got time in between the battle to explain so much things about the reality to Arjuna? We still don't have an answer!! Isn't it? When I was searching and discovering about this the only answer what I was getting was "Krishna's Maya".Many people out there have an opinion that the whole battleground came to a still when Krishna started to preach the essence of gita or his message to Arjuna. It may seem quite confounding about all these raising doubts within us. But more importantly what matters to us more is the message. Sri krishna's message or upadesha to

Arjuna was just not to fight in the outer materialistic war but it was to fight with his own inner world of conflict. While the kauravas represent the bad side of our mind, pandavas the good side!! Though the bad ones try to overpower us all the time in the beginning, there is a voice which is always heard from inside us. The voice from the superconsciousness(representing krishna) to take on the good side and follow the right path(The path of Dharma).We must always remember that whenever this side of goodness(pandavas) or dharma declines there is an inner consciousness (Sri Krishna) to remind us to take on the good side and act according to dharma(what seems as right) as gita says,

Yada yada hi dharmasya glanir bhavati bharatha abhyuttanam adharmasya tadatmanam srjamyaham.

"Whenever there is a downfall of dharma and adharma prevails, I reincarnate myself on this abode for the wellbeing of mankind." With

all these essence of Bhagavadgita, let's start following dharma

by spreading love to the entire universe and being compassionate towards each other.

THE STORY OF GOOD PUNYA

Once upon a time there was a guru living in the southern part of India.Many of the students used to live with him in his ashram and were getting education under him. Once the guru and his disciples were in a discussion. During that time the disciples asked the guru that they had planned to go on a pilgrimage to Varanasi to take a holy dip in the river Ganga so that all their bad karmas(Papas) gets washed away and they could earn good punya by it. So they asked the guru about his decision for allowing them to go on for the pilgrimage. The guru thought on for a while and smiled and said that they could go for the pilgrimage.Seeing the strange smile on the guru's face, the disciples were surprised and said him that they had heard people saying that all their bad papas gets washed away by visiting and taking a holy dip in Ganga river, and asked the guru whether their pilgrimage could be beneficial for that? Then the guru again smiled and started to explain, "See, indeed by visiting to Varanasi and taking a holy dip in the ganga river, all your papas(bad
karmas) gets washed away and you get punya. But those bad karmas which leave your body goes and attaches to the tamarind
tree situated close to the banks of the river. And as soon as you come out of the river, they come back and gets attached with

you again". Now the disciples were shocked and asked guru,"O
revered one, then how can we get rid of our papas(bad karmas)
permanently and prevent them from attaching to us again? ".

For this the guru further replied, " See, to get rid of your bad karmas(papas), you need not go to a pilgrimage to take a dip in
Ganga river. Instead start helping and loving the people around
you. Start being compassionate towards the society around
you. In this way all your bad karmas(papas)gets washed away
from you permanently and you starting gaining punya(good deed) and becoming pure from within". What a great story indeed!! God resides everywhere, so let's start serving the God residing around us in the suffering and needy ones.

RELAXATION TECHNIQUES

Relaxation is a constant endeavour that lies somewhere between effort and non effort.One needs to practice it with skill to get truly relaxed. Yoga is one such skill which helps to relax the body completely both physically as well as mentally. It helps in relaxing the muscles of body as well as mind by a practice known as "Conscious relaxation". In Yoga relaxation always happens by breath. There is a significant relation between mind, body and breath.As hatha yoga describes:

" Chale vate chalam chittam nischale nischalam bhavet
Yogi stanutvamapnothi tatho vayum nirodhayet"

When Prana moves, chitta the mental force moves and when prana stops the mental force stops. Now breath is the one which regulates the movement of prana and hence inturn our chitta or thoughts. Now when we see most of the relaxation techniques in yoga, it almost happens through Shavasana Or Corpse pose.

Though you can sit and relax but I would say sitting always is good when you go for meditation as it focusses on keeping spine straight as well as channeling energies.In relaxation techniques as we want to relax both body and mind completely it is better to practice with Shavasana. So what is Shavasana? It is the posture in which we rest our ten senses.We have never actually discovered who we are!! In a pure sense, we are not the body though we have a body and use it as our temporary home.The body in which we are residing temporarily is a corpse and we are the light dwelling within that corpse.In shavasana we tend to move away from our identification with the body.Knowing this experimentally, through systematic relaxation, is a profound step towards inner peace. Coming to the grosser level shavasana makes the work of the heart easier as it is line with the gravity. Also the heart is in same line with the rest of the body. So it need not pump blood against the gravity as in cases of sitting or standing and thus making its work easier. The field of gravity also creates a subtle tone in the muscles that support your posture. In shavasana, the effect of gravity on these postural muscles is neutralized because the body is completely supported by the floor. This relieves muscle fatigue, allowing you to relax more deeply and making you aware of the dynamic forces acting on your muscles throughout the day. Breathing is also profoundly changed when you rest in shavasana. Muscles attached to the bones of the rib cage, which normally assist in breathing can be relaxed. They rest while contractions of the diaphragm produce a smooth, steady rhythm that calms the nervous system. Tense muscles in the abdominal wall or rib cage that resist deep, diaphragmatic breathing can be gradually relaxed as well. Psychologically, shavasana also calms down the mind and brings balance in nervous system by keeping body still and relaxed. Hence the practice of shavasana forms an important aspect and has been highlighted in almost all the yogic relaxation techniques.But whatever the yogic postures or relaxation techniques, it should be always done under the guidance of a yoga guru or teacher.Keeping that in mind, let's discuss about the relaxation techniques in the further chapters!!

THE MESSAGE OF SWAMI VIVEKANANDA

Swami Vivekananda is an iconic figure in the modern Indian history. In particular he was a key figure in the introduction of Vedantha and Yoga to the Western world.Though he lived only for thirty-nine years, he worked tirelessly to revive the glory of India.Our Prime Minister Shri Narendra Modi is a follower of Swami Vivekananda. His early life has been influenced by the life and works of this spiritual master. Now you may ask me what makes him so much influential? The answer is simple, it's just his life and the message he gave to the world through his life. He advocated on the unity of religions and harmony among them. He always said that the purpose of every individual irrespective of religion was just to spread humanity and serve the mankind. Swami Vivekananda believed that India is the blessed punyabhumi, the "land of virtue".. the land where humanity has attained its highest towards generosity, towards purity, towards calmness, above all, the land of introspection and of spirituality - it is India. " He also always believed in the strength of the youth in nations. He advised the youth to imbibe the strength of spirituality in the youth in making India stand apart at the highest portion in terms of development. He realized that India's strength lies in spirituality, "The Indian nation cannot be killed. Deathless it stands, and it will stand so long as that spirit shall remain as the background,so long as her people do not give up their spirituality". Swamiji also stressed for the rejuvenation of India. And he said that it was possible only when we start believing and understanding our ancient civilization and deep spirituality. Intractable problems of today can be dealt better if principles of spirituality were applied to these.In Swamiji's messages lies the secret of character building and nation building. They are as relevant today as they were in his lifetime. He always believed in the concept of "Universal Religion".He stresses that ,"Upon the banner of every religion soon be written … 'Help and not fight','Assimilation and not Destruction','Harmony and peace and not Dissension'.

If there is anyone who can claim credit that Yoga is scientific, rational and therefore universal, it's Vivekananda. Vivekananda

also laid great emphasis on four Yogas, namely, Bhakti, Karma,

Jnana and Raja Yoga. Each of these classes pertains to a specic

way of attaining the ultimate goal of life – mukti or salvation –

through meticulous and sincere practice.In relation to Yoga he

once famously said, "All this bringing of the mind into a higher

state of vibration is included in one word in Yoga-Samadhi".He

believed that Youth should practise Yoga to fulfill their physical, mental,intellectual and spiritual quests and thus making them reach to higher standards and thus strive for the development of nation.The common error in all ethical systems as well as our education has been the failure of teaching the means by which man could refrain from doing evil under instinctive compulsion. The solution: controlling our nature through the path of yoga. With this end in view, Swamiji thought of a universal way acceptable to all: yoga. To the worker, it is a union between man and whole of humanity, to the mystic, between his higher and lower selves, to the lover, a union between himself and God of love, to the philosopher, it is a union of all existence. Swamiji asserted that each soul is potentially divine with omnipotence and omniscience, awaiting manifestation. We can realise the same through selfless service, assimilation of wisdom through deeper introspection, devotion to the Almighty or some special psychophysical practice.To Swamiji, selfless service was a unique path for Self-realisation. Swami Vivekananda compared human mind with that of a monkey which is always restless and relentlessly wants to do something. In the same way

human
mind always wants to get outside through the channels of the
body. So he stressed on the practice of Ekagratha or dhyana i.e.
concentration through yoga and thus enhancing the strength of
mind. He always believed that there is no limit to human mind,
the more focussed it is, the more powerful it becomes.
Throughout his life, Swami Vivekananda strived to uplift the
plight of women, in particular Indian women.He always believed in the gender quality and propounded on it,"When people are discussing as to what man and woman can do, always the same mistake is made. They think they show man at his best because he can fight, for instance, and undergo tremendous physical exertion; and this is pitted against the physical weakness and non-combating quality of woman. This is unjust. Woman is as courageous as man. Each is equally good in his of her way. What man can bring up a child with such patience, endurance, and love as the woman can? The one has developed the power of doing; the other, the power of suffering. If woman cannot act, neither can man suffer. The whole universe is one of perfect balance."
When we speak about wealth, it gets spoilt when it is kept over for a long time without using it.In the same way Swamiji believed that Indian wealth i.e.Yoga and spirituality should be expanded and exchanged with the Western philosophy. Then only there would be a growth in philosophy and yogic system by bringing about

manifestation within each of us and also with our approach towards them. In one of the letter written to his follower Alasinga perumal, Vivekananda writes, "The whole world requires Light. It is expectant! India alone has that Light, not in magic, mummery, and charlatanism, but in the teaching of the glories of the spirit of real religion — of the highest spiritual truth. That is why the Lord has preserved the race through all its vicissitudes unto the present day. Now the time has come. Have faith that you are all, my brave lads, born to do great things! Let not the barks of puppies frighten you — no, not even the thunderbolts of heaven — but stand up and work!

With these messages of Swami Vivekananda lets start marching
towards making India as “Vishwaguru” to the entire world as
dreamt by him!!

WHY ONE NEEDS TO CHANT AUM

We all would have been probably heard this chanting atleast once in our lifetime.It has become a means of beginning and ending aspect for those who are in the practice of yoga. Yogis are always seen chanting this repeatedly with a certain amount of vibration. We all would have seen in movies, whenever a person sits for penance or meditation it can be depicted only when he starts chanting omkara. Now we can say how much omkara has become familiar with all of us in our day to day lives. Omkara should always be set apart from the religious point of view, it should never be seen as a posession of just Hindu religion but instead should become an asset in one's daily routine to make oneself pure and calm within. Though it has originated from Hindu Dharma, it always represents the nature of the universe. It comprises of the cosmic energy that runs the whole world. Hence anything connected with the universe and creation should always be viewed away from religious point. This symbol AUM consists of three letters of which each letter symbolizes the cyclical nature of Nature itself, as a movement from birth to death. Of its three syllables, it has four parts:

'A' representing the beginning of a life cycle and the impetus of creativity, 'U' representing the middle of a life cycle and the sustaining of it, 'M' representing the end of a life cycle

and the destruction of it, and a silent pause where sound itself dissolves
into space before the cycle begins again.In Hindu cosmology, Aum is a bija mantra, or sacred seed sound, which created all other sounds and vibrations in our universe. Aum was the original vibration that rippled through pure enlightened awareness, creating the complicated patterns of our individual consciousness. The analogy in Mundaka Upanishad describes that Om is the bow; the soul is the arrow; and Brahman is the target.The target is attained by an unerring man. One should become one with the target just like an arrow. This is to become one with the imperishable by eliminating the ideas of the body, ego, prana.Hence being the self with nothing less than union with the absolute. Further mandukya upanishad describes omkara as the syllable of past, present and future. Patanjali yoga sutras also defined omkara as "tasya vachakah pranavah", thus defining omkara as Shiva. It also describes that Sadhana is required for this realisation of omkara Or Ishwara,"Tajjapah tadarthabhavanam" which defines that mental repitition of Aum should be carried out while dwelling on its meaning". During my childhood days I used to visit an old Shiva temple in my native near Tamil nadu.Many of these old shiva temples near Tamil nadu are very famous not just because of their majestic size but also because of their holyness and a vast history they carry along with them. Here in this temple,I always used to hear the omkara chanting near the Lord. Maybe they would have played that from a voice recorder. But the pleasant feeling it used to give to
the entire atmosphere inside the Garbha gudi was exceptional.Except the light near the moorthi in garbha

gudi, there used to be no light inside temple, I still haven't figured out why though, but in that darkness the light shining with brightness near the Lord along with this omkara chanting would make anyone stay there.The priest after finishing pooja when he used to come to us to give us flowers and vibhooti was always found to be sweating. Even during a cold atmosphere around,this used to happen. Many people used to say this as power of the Shiva inside and for the same reason many say no one can sleep inside Shiva temple for a night for all alone throughout. But at a definite point at that time in that silent atmosphere, it made me understand that there is some power running around in this world which tends to come out at certain places or instances where it finds suitable probably favourable conditions.

This made me feel that whether God or Ishvara exists or not we

don't know, but the power of omkara will make the power behind universe to come out in any atmosphere if it is felt and chanted or listened to by coming across these events. Omkar, pronounced in its correct method, arouses and transforms every atom in the physical body, setting up new vibrations and conditions, and awakening the sleeping power of the body. The chanting of AUM drives away all worldly thoughts and removes distractions. It is very powerful. If you are depressed, chant AUM for 10 minutes, you will be filled with new vigour and strength. Chanting of AUM gives energy. Continuous practice of Omkar helps in improving the brain capacity and memory. Our capacity to grasp any knowledge increases. Our mind becomes more active and we are able to take decisions quickly. Our brain has 14000 centres. However we are only utilizing 208 centres or just 2% of the brain. The other 98% of the brain remains unused. Chanting of Omkar stimulates these sleeping brain centres. Just 5 minutes of Omkar chanting gives calmness and relaxation to our body and mind. As we inhale deeply while chanting AUM, we take more oxygen in, improving the capacity of lungs. Chanting of AUM improves confidence level and prepares us to face the adverse circumstances of life. AUM removes nervousness and fears from the mind. Chanting of Omkar before bed gives sound sleep. The problems of Insomnia and fearful dreams are cured by AUM chanting. Omkara can be chanted either slowly or fastly. Each method is as good as the other and you must experiment yourself to find out your own preference. If chanted quickly, then it is a powerful method to synchronize it with the heartbeat. In this manner you feel AUM resonating throughout the whole body in tune with the natural heart rate. If AUM is chanted slowly, it can be made to last many seconds, depending on the capacity of the individual. There should be a definite pronunciation of each of the syllables 'A', 'U' and 'M', with a gradual transition of one to another. 'A' is pronounced as 'a' in 'palm', 'U' is pronounced as 'ooo', and 'M' is pronounced as a humming sound by closing the lips 'mmmmmmm'. The sound of 'A' should start at the navel, 'U' from the chest and 'M' from brain (head). The sound should be generated from the navel and taken up very slowly to the top of the head with the closing sound of 'M'. 'A' is pronounced by opening the mouth slightly, without touching the tongue to the pallets of the mouth, 'U' is pronounced by opening the mouth in a beak shape, like whistling, the tongue touching the back of the lower teeth slightly, 'M' is pronounced by closing the mouth and simply producing the humming sound (mmmmmmmm). All the three sounds should be continuous and in rhythm, like the water pouring continuously. Just like the ringing of a bell the sound and vibrations are heard for a long time, called 'ninaad'. In the same way AUM should be chanted, with the 'M' sound leaving its vibration. This causes a vibration in our body AUM is the cosmic sound.

AUM is everywhere. AUM is in the rotation of the earth, all the other planets, stars. Everything in the cosmos is in motion and

constantly producing a sound. That constant humming sound is
AUM. The motion creates speed, the speed creates sound and energy. The universe is so huge that we are unable to perceive it.
AUM sound is continuous in the universe but we are so tiny in
the universe that we are unable to hear this sound. By chanting
of AUM we are creating the sound of AUM and trying to create
the vibration within our body. The symbol of Omkar has 4 parts, each part corresponds with a particular stage in human
life. According to Indian philosophy the life of a human being
undergoes 4 stages. The rst part, the half circle denotes the rst
stage of human life until we nish our education. The rst stage
is from birth up to the age of 25 until we nish our education.
This stage is called Brahmacharya. The second part, or the second half circle, represents the second stage of human life. The
second stage is from the age of 25 up to the age of 50 years. This
stage is called the grihastha ashram. In this stage, the human
being plays the role of a householder, spouse, parent, employee,
businessman etc. The third part, the full circle represents

the
third stage of human life. After the age of 50, the third stage
starts, when the children are grown up and are able to take care
of themselves. The responsibilities of family are much reduced.
In this stage of life, man should turn his focus into his social responsibilities by sharing and caring with the society in various
ways. This stage is called Vanprastha and it lasts up to the age of
75. The last stage of human life is from 75 to 100 years. The children are grown up now and they don't need help anymore, one is
free from responsibility. At that stage you have to be satised
and that is the complete nature of life. One should divert all attention to becoming spiritual. This stage is called sannyasa. The
bindu (dot) in the Omkar symbol represents this fourth part of
human life. Where the man works towards his liberation, by
keeping one pointed focus on God. The path of bindu will lead
our way to god.
With these discussion lets start chanting omkara not just as a practice but throughout our day whenever we are free in our
busy schedule of life and thus make ourselves and our

souls pure
and thus channeling the pure cosmic energy within us.

OMKARA MEDITATION

Nadhanusandhana is a form of sound based breathing technique which has been propounded in Hatha yoga text by Swami Swatmarama. "Nada" refers to the "sound" and "Anusandhana" refers to the "connecting".Hence "Connecting to the sound"forms the major basis for Nadhanusandhana technique as such.

TECHNIQUE: It involves four stages as such:

1)ARAMBHA AVASTHA Pranava(OM) should be chanted with three Matras(prolonged intonations) to destroy all his former sins. At this stage one accomplishes the Arambha Avastha and one starts to perspire. At this point one should rub it well with the hands. The trembling of body may also occur sometimes.

2) GHATA AVASTHA Then follows the Ghata Avastha , which

is acquired by constant practice of the suppression of breath.

When a perfect union takes place between Prana and Apana,

Manas and Buddhi, or Jivatman and Paratman, without opposition it is called Ghata Avastha. Day by day the duration should be increased to finally reach 3 hours. He should also practice kevala kumbhaka once in a day. By cesssation of breath, one

starts to practise pratyahara. He starts to detach himself

from the material objects he percieves through his senses.Whatever
one percieves through his senses, he should consider them as Atman.At this stage, the yogi or Sadhaka starts to acquire Siddhis
or supernatural powers which the yogi should always consider it as obstacles in the true path of yoga and should never get deviated towards them.He should not excercise these powers before
anyone whomsoever. He should always live his life as an ordinary man to conceal his powers and carry on with his further
practice. Thus one who constantly engaged in yogic practises
passes the Ghata avastha.

3) PARICHAYA AVASTHA With such constant practice, one attains the third stage of Parichaya avastha. Vayu or breath
through such focussed practise pierces the kundalini, along with agni and enters sushumna, uninterrupted. When this happens the yogi acquires the power of Kriya shakti and the vayu along with agni pierces through the six Chakras and the yogi reaches the secure condition of Parichaya. Then the Yogi can free himself from the karmas by by the Pranava(OM). At this stage of yoga,one can practise "Kaya vyuha", a mystical process of arranging various skandhas of the body and taking various bodies also known as parakaya pravesha to free oneself from the previous karmas without the necessity of being reborn. At this stage let the yogi practise the ve dharanas i.e.,concentrating on the
ve chakras starting from Mooladhara to Vishuddhi by

which command over ve elements of nature is gained and fear of being injured by anyone of them is removed.

4) NISHPATTI AVASTHA This is the fourth stage. Through the graduated and steady practice of Nadhanusandhana,the yogi reaches the stage of Nishpatti Avastha, the stage of consummation. The yogi having destroyed all the seeds of karma drinks the nectar of immortality. He enjoys the bliss of samadhi. He is free from hunger, thirst, pain,disease, old age and death. He is no longer in need of any yogic practice. He is entitled to get liberation. A Yogic student will automatically experience all these Avasthas one by one as he advances in his systematic, regular practices. An impatient student cannot experience any of these Avasthas through occasional practices. Care should be taken in the observance of yogic diet(natural and light food i.e.sattvic diet)and Brahmacharya. Though this practice may seem bit highly spiritual and above a normal man's belief, we should never stop the practice as only at the higher stages of practice we tend to start understanding these experiences deep within us. Even though if one may not experience these things,

there
is nothing to lose as it has many physical and mental benets at the beginner's stages. As the chanting of Omkara itself
removes all our unwanted thoughts and makes a person calm
and relaxed as discussed earlier. So let's inculcate the practice
of Nadhanusandhana in our lives to make it more happier and
worthful!!

YOGA NIDRA

Nidra is always termed as "sleep". For every human being sleep is very much essential. It's the one which makes a man feel refreshed mentally and physically. But in this today's so called "Rat race", are we sleeping properly is the question?The answer is may be not.Yoga always speaks about consciouness i.e.being conscious in the karma you do making realise its effect. In the same way, can we also do with the sleep ?

Of course and hence Yoga nidra is also referred to as " conscious sleep".The origin of Yoga nidra has been said to be from tantric cult. So now let's move on to this technique of practice as such.

Outline Of The Practice :

1.Preparation for the practice:By lying down in shavasana.

2)Resolution:It should be always non-materialistic.

3.Rotation of consciousness:Right side of body to left side of body then towards back and coming to forward aspect of body and atlast towards the major parts of the body.

4.Awareness of breath: depends on the variation or type of yoga

nidra practised.
5.Awareness of feelings and sensations: depends on the variation or type of yoga nidra practised.
4.Visualisation: depends on the variation or type of yoga nidra
practised.
5.Ending the practise.

Basically Yoga nidra has five variations. This was just an outline
of all the variations together. In each variation there are different procedures within these outlines to be done. Let's move on
to the first variation as such:
1.Yoga Nidra 1:
Preparation
Relaxation:Body/OM Resolution
Rotation of consciousness: Right side,left side, Back,front, major parts of body.
Breathing:Counting breaths with navel, chest, throat and nostril awareness;each 27 to 1.
Image visualisation:Introductory.
Resolution
Finish
Alternation short practises-As an interlude at work. As a prelude to sleep.

2)Yoga Nidra 2:
Preparation
Relaxation:Anthar mouna
Resolution
Rotation of consciousness: Right side,left side, Back, front,

major parts of body.
Body/Floor awareness
Breathing:Breathing throat to navel:54 to 1 or 27 to 1.
Awareness of sensations: Heaviness/lightness, cold/heat, pain/pleasure,
Inner space :chidakasha
Visualisation:Park/temple
Resolution
Finish
Alternative visualisation: Mountain,floating body, well/ocean.

3)Yoga Nidra 3:
Preparation
Relaxation:Anthar mouna
Resolution
Rotation of consciousness:Right side,left side,Back, front, major parts of body.
Skin awareness
Breathing: Mentally,alternate nostril: 108 to 1 time without closing nostrils.
Inner space :chidakasha
Visualisation:Eyebrow centre/OM
Resolution
Finish
Alternative visualisation: Golden egg, climbing the sacred mountain.

4) Yoga Nidra 4:
Preparation
Relaxation:Anthar mouna
Resolution

Rotation of consciousness:Right side,left side,Back, front, major parts of body.
Skin awareness
Breathing: Mentally, alternate nostril: 108 to 1 time without closing nostrils.
Inner space :Chidakasha
Visualisation:Eyebrow centre/OM
Resolution
Finish
Alternative visualisation: Golden egg, climbing the sacred mountain.

5)Yoga Nidra 5:
Preparation
Relaxation:Antar mouna
Resolution
Rotation of consciousness: Right side,left side,Back,front, major parts of body.
Breathing: Mentally, alternate nostril: 108 to 1 time without closing nostrils.
Visualisation:Eyebrow centre/OM/
Ocean/Temple.
Resolution
Finish
Alternative visualisation: Psychic centers, Psychic symbols,eyebrow center/Om, Rapid images, Transparent body,
aura,golden egg.

Yog nidra should never be seen as normal sleep. It is a going-to sleep stage which not just involves physical and mental rest but goes one step forward to the deep subconscious level. Hence all the hidden emotions within a man comes out and eradicates. Thus making him more peaceful and calm within. It is said that a single hour of Yoga nidra is as restful as four hours of conventional sleep.If diseases progress in the psychosomatic path,Yoga nidra is always found to act or relieve it by the reverse direction i.e.somatopsychic way. Hence it has been found to be very much beneficial in cases of insomnia and ischemic heart diseases. So why waiting? Let's begin our practice of yogic way of sleep in our day to day lives!!

ZEN MEDITATION

Now let me start discussing you with some of my views caught up with while coming across Zen meditation.
Zen meditation is a form of meditation that evolved from parts of India and China. It is a part of Chinese spirituality and held in Zen seat of buddhism. "Zen" is a Japanese word translated from the Chinese word "chan" which means "meditation". Being aware of your body as well as your breath is the basis of this meditation.

History: Coming to the historical background of this meditation as such, Bodhidharma is the legendary founder of Zen meditation who brought it in China. Legend Bodhidharma, a South Indian king, who travelled all the way to China to spread real Buddhism, introduced the concept "Zen".
Now what are the basic concepts of Zen ? Let's go on with them as such:
1. The first basic concept which even I have been stressing on
alot times earlier is compassion. Zen meditation stresses that
along with wisdom, compassion forms an important aspect i.e.,
believing on oneness of all the living beings. This forms an important aspect in removing hatred from oneself about

others.

2.The next comes the concept of conditioned arising or Interdependent co-arising.It has been also said as "causal nexus".This can be easily said as the process of chain reaction or theory of cause and effect as such.It stated that whatever the physiological and psychological phenomena that make up an individual's existence are interdependant and mutually condition each other.

3) After that comes the concept of "No mind".Perceiving the

objects as they are present. It might not be just with the case of

objects but can also be with the circumstances or events.

1. Next comes the concept of " No Self".It apprehends the concept of impersonality of existence that means existence is just an

influx of arising and moving away of physical and mental phenomena and there is no constant individual self or ego.

2. Lastly comes the important concept i.e.,"Wisdom".The central notion of Zen says that experienced inherent wisdom cannot be conveyed by concepts or intellectual terms.The actual moment of wisdom comes by our insight into emptiness that comes by one's own personal experience.

After coming across some of he basic concepts of Zen, let's move

on to the technique as such. The procedure is simple as such and

just focusses mainly on the posture and stillness.

1. Find an adequately lit room with a comfortable temperature. Take a medium sized cushion traditionally called "Zafu" and place it on the mat that you will sit on.

2. The cushion ensures that the hips are elevated, the knees face downwards towards the ground.Wear loose airy, and comfortable clothing and sit on the cushion in either the Full lotus
pose(Padmasana)/Half lotus pose as such.

SITTING STRAIGHT

3. For the Full lotus pose, Both of your feet on the opposite
thigh;on the both sides.

4. A Half lotus pose is when you place either of your ankles on
the opposite thigh.

5. If sitting like this is uncomfortable, a kneeling position or
sitting in a backless bench will also do, ideally the sitting position is recommended.

6. Make sure your back is erect and upright.Keep the body erect
and balanced,not too relaxed or tensed.

EYE GAZE

7. In Zen meditation,the eyes are not completely closed.

8. Partially closed eyes help you stay alert and avoid drowsiness.Keep your eyes half closed and direct your gaze diagonally lower towards the ground.

9. You don't have to focus anything particular, ideally it is best to sit in front of a wall to avoid distractions.

Basic Zen technique: 1)At this point begin counting your breath, count on inhalation as one, then exhalation as two, and continue your breaths until you reach count 10.

10.After reaching 10,at that point return to count with 1 with
the next inhalation. If at any point you are caught with

mental distraction and loose your count, gently without passing any judgement return to 1 and start over. That's it, continue for the entire duration of meditation.

Intermediate Zen technique: Follow all the steps for the basic Zen meditation technique except the count i.e., a complete inhalation and exhalation cycle should be counted as 1. So you will do 10 full cycles of inhalation and exhalation before returning to 1. You can also increase time upto 30-40 minutes.

Advanced Zen technique: Follow all the steps of basic Zen meditation technique, except for the counting of breath, just let "Be in the breath" and involves following the inhalations and exhalations of the breath with the mind's eye only.This is known as "Following the breath".Never try to jump to this step too soon. Just try to first build your concentration and focus by basic and intermediate practices. After that one must slowly get into the advanced practice.

Set your Mind:As you sit in meditative posture and breathe,thoughts buried deep in your unconsciousness mind are bound to resurface and play around in your head.

Do not pursue those thoughts either by giving into them/avoid them as they will only affect you more. Just let them pass like a flowing river. Ideally a beginner should meditate for 15-30 minutes.

There is also other two concepts which have been mentioned in Zen meditation which are as follows:

1)Koan:A phrase from a teaching of realisation. Koans are not the nonsensical riddles that need to be solved rather they are the subtle teachings of one's own life. They can never be solved by logic but their meaning can only be intuited by personal experience. Koans are used as meditative subjects. Students who have sufficiently settled their wandering states of mind may be given(where there is no teacher available)themselves to select a koan to meditate upon.

2)Shikantaza:Next comes the concept called Shikantaza.In Japanese it refers to "just sitting".It is said to be non-reactive attention that neither pursues nor reflects thoughts, sensations,etc., but rather gives alert detached attention to whatever arises in and vanishes from the consciousness, whether inside or outside your body. It is being fully aware that your body is sitting. Lastly going on to the breathing part as such, breathe quietly through your nose during zazen.As you relax, proper posture will allow you to naturally start abdominal breathing.This occurs when your abdomen moves outwards to inhale and inwards to exhale, rather than breathing with the chest. Abdominal breathing in turn promotes further relaxed awareness.Do not try to control your breathing. Let it come and go naturally.

Coming to the benefits of Zen meditation as such many research papers tell us that it helps us in providing relaxation

in many brain regions particularly in the frontal cortex and enhancing alpha and theta waves of brain activity particularly

theta activity as it involves "openness to experience".As it involves major effects on frontal cortex it protects oneself from cognitive decline usually associated with age and enhance antioxidant activity. From a clinical point of view Zen meditation was found to reduce stress and blood pressure and found to be efficacious in variety of clinical conditions as such. The basic hindrance in a person's life for realisation according to the Zen concept is that although we have never experienced the present moment we assume that we know about it.

NOW i.e., the present moment is here and unknown-the unpredictable meeting that is Life. Moment by moment each one is unique and unrepeatable, once occuring chance to discover NOW. So let's start and get going and practice Zen meditation to discover our present and beautiful moments of Life!!

NADHANUSANDANA

Nadhanusandhana is a form of sound based breathing technique which has been propounded in Hatha yoga text by Swami Swatmarama. "Nada" refers to the "sound" and "Anusandhana" refers to the "connecting".Hence "Connecting to the sound"forms the major basis for Nadhanusandhana technique as such.

TECHNIQUE: It involves four stages as such:

1)ARAMBHA AVASTHA Pranava(OM) should be chanted with three Matras(prolonged intonations) to destroy all his former sins. At this stage one accomplishes the Arambha Avastha and one starts to perspire. At this point one should rub it well with the hands. The trembling of body may also occur sometimes.

2) GHATA AVASTHA Then follows the Ghata Avastha , which

is acquired by constant practice of the suppression of breath.

When a perfect union takes place between Prana and Apana,

Manas and Buddhi, or Jivatman and Paratman, without opposition it is called Ghata Avastha. Day by day the duration should be increased to finally reach 3 hours. He should also practice kevala kumbhaka once in a day. By cessation of breath, one starts to practise pratyahara. He starts to detach himself from the material objects he percieves through his senses.Whatever one percieves through his senses, he should consider them as Atman.At this stage, the yogi or Sadhaka starts to acquire Siddhis or supernatural powers which the yogi should always consider it as obstacles in the true path of yoga and should never get deviated towards them.He should not excercise these powers before anyone whomsoever. He should always live his life as an ordinary man to conceal his powers and carry on with his further practice. Thus one who is constantly engaged in these yogic practises passes the Ghata avastha.

3) PARICHAYA AVASTHA With such constant practice, one attains the third stage of Parichaya avastha. Vayu or breath through such focussed practise pierces the kundalini, along with agni and enters sushumna, uninterrupted. When this happens, the yogi acquires the power of Kriya shakti and the vayu along with agni pierces through the six Chakras and the yogi reaches the secure condition of Parichaya. Then the Yogi can free himself from the karmas by the Pranava(OM). At this stage of yoga,one can practise "Kaya vyuha", a mystical process of arranging various skandhas of the body and taking various bodies also known as parakaya pravesha to free oneself from the previous karmas without the necessity of being reborn. At this stage let the yogi practise the five dharanas i.e.,concentrating on the five chakras starting from Mooladhara to Vishuddhi by which command over five elements of nature is gained and fear of being injured by anyone of them is removed.

4) NISHPATTI AVASTHA This is the fourth stage. Through the graduated and steady practice of Nadhanusandhana,the yogi
reaches the stage of Nishpatti Avastha, the stage of

consummation. The yogi having destroyed all the seeds of karma drinks the nectar of immortality. He enjoys the bliss of samadhi. He is free from hunger, thirst, pain,disease, old age and death. He is no longer in need of any yogic practice. He is entitled to get liberation. A Yogic student will automatically experience all these
Avasthas one by one as he advances in his systematic, regular
practices. An impatient student cannot experience any of these
Avasthas through occasional practices. Care should be taken
in the observance of yogic diet(natural and light food i.e.sattvic diet)and Brahmacharya. Though this practice may seem bit
highly spiritual and above a normal man's belief, we should never stop the practice as only at the higher stages of practice
we tend to start understanding these experiences deep within
us. Even though if one may not experience these things, there
is nothing to lose as it has many physical and mental benets at the beginner's stages. As the chanting of Omkara itself
removes all our unwanted thoughts and makes a person calm
and relaxed as discussed earlier. So let's inculcate the practice
of Nadhanusandhana in our lives to make it more happier and
worthful!!

VIPASSANA MEDITATION

"Peace comes from within, Do not seek it without".

-

Buddha

As the above quote says, the technique of Vipassana meditation also known as "Insight meditation"is simple, practical way to achieve real piece of mind and to lead a happy, useful life. Vipassana means"to see things as they really are" and the technique is a logical process of mental purication by self observation. Vipassana is one of the most ancient meditation techniquestechniques discovered in India 2500 years ago by Gautama Buddha, the essence of what he practised and taught during his 45 years of teaching. Few centuries after Buddha, Vipassana had disappeared from India. In our time Vipassana has been reintroduced by Sir Satyanarayan Goenka. It has been mostly practised as a ten days residential course under the guidance of a qualied teacher. During

these
ten days, the sadhakas remain within the course site, free from
outside distractions. Buddha also recommemds that for successful meditation, one must resort to Palibodha meaning cutting down impediments or disturbing elementselements which
try to distract him from the path of enlightment.
TECHNIQUE: 1)During the rst 3 days students learn how to
calm and focus the mind with the help of the breath.They focus on their natural ow of breath that comes and leaves the nostril. This is said to enhance the concentration of a person and
a tool for penetratinh self-analysis. This process of developing
concentration through focus on breath is known as Anapana.
2) On the fourth day they learn the practice of vipassana meditation itself. Instead of focussing on one point, they tend
to move their focus thought their body i.e.shifting focus from
head to toes and again focussing from toes to head. Trying to observe the sensations such as heat, pressure, cold, etc., whether
pleasant or unpleasantunpleasant, every sensation is to be observed and accepted dispassionately. This causes the supresses
or deeply hidden emotions to come out which are the source of
mental agitation. These hidden emotions come out

accompanied by physical sensations.The meditators are instructed to give importance only to actual sensations, practicing to percieve it's impermanent nature.

3) The third sub-unit in vipassana is the development of Metta bhavana i.e., to have Universal Love and compassion which we should try to instill throughout and after the process of meditation as such. Love all and hate none. Always one must know that vipassana practice involves 3 phases:

1. Sheela:Right speech, Right action,Right livelihood.
2. Samadhi:Right eort, Right concentration, Right mindfulness.
3. Prajna:Right view, Right resolution. Sheela is the footstep,Samadhi is the way and Prajna is the destination. One must understand that Vipassana is always being joyful from the very beginning of practice, during the journey and joyful at its destination. It's been found in one of the research done by Symbiosis International University that the practice of Vipassana meditation not just reduced stress as such but also brought about an inner transformation and develop intrinsic characteristics from a group of employees practising 10 days of Vipassana meditation.It also showed that it signicantly contributed to their psychological well being and inturn adding meaning to

their lives. Then why waiting? Let's start to begin with the practise of Vipassana in your upcoming days to transform yourselves and be the best!!

TRANSCEDENTAL MEDITATION

Now moving on, the next comes the Transcedental meditation which is a natural and effortless practice by which mind transcends to its nest state of thought. It was founded by Maharshi Mahesh Yogi. Transcends means "to go beyond" i.e., to go beyond materialism and reach Self-realisation.

TECHNIQUE:

1. In Transcedental meditation, the Guidance of a Guru is mandatory.
2. The practise is initiated by a guru wherein he tells a secret mantra to the practitioner.
3. The practitioner repeats the mantra and meditates upon it, without any effort.
4. The longer the duration,the mantra will become a part of the practitioner's mind replacing unnecessary thoughts and the mind becomes calm.
5. In the Transcedental meditation, the duration of meditation should be slowly increased by 10 seconds by repeated series of opening eyes for 5 seconds after each phase of meditation for a particular duration. If one meditates for 10 seconds then he should open his eyes for 3-5 seconds and then again close his eyes and meditate upon mantra for 20 seconds before opening his eyes and so on.The duration of Transcedental meditation is for five days.I personally also tried practised Transcedental

meditation in my college and it instills a sense of calmness within and also refreshes your mind. And coming to the benefits of Transcedental meditation as such it also gives the same benefits as the other by inducing more alpha wave activity in the brain. As the mind
experiences inner states of thought, correspondingly the body settles to deeper states of rest. This produces a state of restful-alertness(Alpha) where the body is in deep state of restfulness while the mind is alert. This state of restfulness-alertness is known to be of greater benefit to body and mind. Unlike other
meditations, Transcedental meditation does not recommend any posture as such. It is just practised while sitting comfortably with eyes closed. But one must always remember that Transcedental meditation should always be practised under the guidance of a guru as he is the one who initiates the mantra.

There have been a lot of commendable researches done on Transcedental meditation which is found to be very much beneficial in cardiovascular disorders. So let's get going and practice this wonderful meditation and as Swamiji says achieve the expansion of happiness throughout this world!!

INSTANT RELAXATION TECHNIQUE(IRT)

Swami Vivekananda emphasized the importance of reducing stress both physically as well as mentally and introduced the concept of Instant Relaxation technique which forms an important part along with other two techniques of Cyclic meditation which I have discussed in my upcoming chapters.Before beginning any of these techniques one must always observe breathing at the tip of nostrils for sometime, the way air comes in and goes out through the nostrils. Then only he must go on with the practice of these three techniques. Coming to Instant Relaxation technique as such, it is an immediate

way of relaxing the body and mind. It is usually practiced at the beginning of the yoga session to perform the yogic poses better and achieve maximum benefits. It has been found to be very much good to relieve pain during yogic sessions and also during prenatal yogic sessions. The principle is to stretch in first phase and then relax which is done in second phase. It works at physical level.

PROCEDURE:

1. Join the legs, heels and toes in shavasana. Arms by the side of the body, palms touching thighs.
2. Tighten the toes and ankle joints.
3. Sensitize the soles.

4. Stretch the calf muscles and tighten.
5. Tighten and pull up the knee caps.
6. Exhale and suck the abdomen.
7.Inhale and expand the chest.
8.Tighten the shoulder region, arms and forearm.
9. Make a st of hand.
10.Tighten neck muscles, facial muscles and squeeze the facial muscles.
11. Exhale and release legs, hands and relax completely.
12. Repeat this again for about 3 rounds to start with, gradually going deeper and longer with the holding of breath and the
muscles.
13.For better results, changing of "OM"kara can also be done at the end of IRT. These vibrations of omkar deep within
the relaxed muscles help in bringing in fresh blood flow and energy to the entire body.

DURATION:Can be practised for 45 seconds to 1 minute.

Who should not practise?

1. As there involves holding of breath, people with hypertension are not advisable to practise IRT.
2. For the same above reason even the people with heart conditions should avoid practsing IRT instead go on with other techniques.
3. As the muscles are pulled tightly, it is also not safe for pregnant women to practice IRT.
3. And also those suffering from fibromyalgia should also avoid it as it involves holding of breath and pulling of muscles.

What do you get by practicing IRT?

Coming to the benefits as such, mainly it is an anytime

practice which calms down the mind by reducing the stress and also prepares the body and mind for the practice of Yoga. Hence you can give a try and practice IRT before beginning with your yoga session and feel the magical change in your yogic practice!!

QUICK RELAXATION TECHNIQUE(QRT)

Next let's move on to the second technique introduced by Swami Vivekananda which is also a part of Cyclic meditation called as Quick Relaxation Technique.Quick relaxation technique is a relaxative procedure that is usually done after standing yoga poses practice. QRT is done best when the cues are given by someone else to help one get maximum benefits. QRT involves 3 phases as such:1. Physical level 2. Mental level 3. Pranic level

TECHNIQUE:

1.Observation of abdominal muscle movements: a)Feel the movement of abdomen:upward and downward. b)Just observe and do not alter the breath for five rounds.

2. Synchronize with breathing: a) With inhalation abdomen bulges up and with exhalation it sinks down. b) Synchronize movement with breathing for five rounds.

3. Breathing with feeling: a) As you inhale,take positive energy from atmosphere around you. b) As you exhale, release all your tiredness and lethargy from body and mind. c) With each inhalation feel energised and with each exhalation feel relaxed.

Who should not practise QRT?

1. People with back injury should avoid QRT as this technique can never be done in sitting posture. It can be

done only if provided the back is well supported and feet touching the floor.

2. In case of Trauma patients who feel uncomfortable to close their eyes this technique can be avoided.

What do I get by the practise of QRT?

There are a lot of benefits involved with the practise of QRT as such as it helps in developing awareness and relaxing the body.Hence let's get going and practise Quick Relaxation technique in our day to day lives!!

DURATION:It can be practised for 3 minutes.

DEEP RELAXATION TECHNIQUE(DRT)

Now let's move on to the last technique which is a part of Cyclic meditation known as Deep relaxation technique. Deep relaxation technique as the name suggests is a deeper and more intense form of relaxation technique.Deep relaxation technique is usually done at the end of the yogic practice.

TECHNIQUE: One should lie down inshavasana. Deep relaxation technique involves 7 phases as such.

These phases have to practised in the same order as follows:

Phase 1: Relaxation of Lower part of body -Each part starting from toes is sensitized and relaxed with the soles of foot,ankles, calf muscles, knees, thighs, buttocks, pelvic region upto the waist.

-To enhance the relaxation of lower part of the body chant 'A'kara and feel vibrations in the lower part of body.

Phase 2:Relaxation of Middle part of body -Shift your awareness to middle part of the body. -Observe and relax the abdomen,

chest, back, hands, arms, neck, shoulder region. To enhance the relaxation of middle part of body chant 'U'kara and feel vibrations in the middle part of body.

Phase 3:Relaxation of Head Region: -Shift your awareness

to the head region.

-Observe and relax the chin, cheeks, teeth, gums, tongue, eyes, ears, eyebrows, eyelashes, forehead and head. Chant

'M'kara to enhance the relxation and feel vibration to enhance the relaxatio at the head region.

Phase 4:Relaxation of Whole body: -Observe the whole body from toes to head and relax.

-Chant the "AUM" in single breath. Feel the resonance throughout the body.

Phase 5:Visualisation of body: -Slowly come out of the body consciousness.

-Visualise the body lying on the ground, completely collapsed.

Phase 6:Visualisation of the Sky: -Imagine the vast beautiful blue sky.

-Expand your awareness and merge yourself into beautiful sky. Enjoy the innite bliss, a state of science.

Phase 7:Ending the practice: -Slowly come back to bodily consciousness. -Gently move your whole body little. Feel the lightness, alterness and movement of

energy throughout the body.

DURATION:Deep Relaxation Technique can be practised for around 6-10 minutes.

Who should not practise DRT?

-People with any back injury should avoid practise of DRT

-Also people with severe acidity can also avoid DRT as the procedure involved lying down for a long time and the person may feel uncomfortable during the practice.

What do I get by the practice of DRT?

As DRT involves a long duration lying down with

awareness,this beautiful technique gives a room for connecting with 'you' and helps in finding answers to many unanswered questions. It helps to completely learn to surrender and try and connect with the 'soul'. Along with the other two techniques it has many physical benefits such as reducing stress, reducing blood pressure and helping in combating the daily challenges and riddles throughout our lives!!

CYCLIC MEDITATION

It has been also referred to as SMET(Self Management of Excessive Tension)which has its origin from the Mandukya Upanishad.Cyclic meditation is a type of meditation which involves a series of successive stimulation and relaxation to remove stress from deeper layers of consciousness.The very basis
of Cyclic Meditation has been taken from Mandukya upanishad where the essence of sadhana has been described.

PRAYER: Laye sambhodayet chittam vikshiptam samayetpunah
sakashayam vijaniyat sampraptam na chalayet
It states that "in a state of oblivion(state of being unaware) awaken the mind,when agitated pacify it, if the mind
has attained perfect state of equilibrium do not disturb it again".

SIGNIFICANCE:
1. Stimulate the awareness and awaken the mind.
2. Calm down the distracted mind.
3. Each stimulation removed the lethargy and stagnation.
4. These relaxes the deeper layers of Human personality.

TYPES OF AWARENESS INVOLVED IN THE PRACTICE OF CYCLIC MEDITATION:

1. Surface Awareness
2. One-pointed Awareness
3. Linear Awareness
4. 3D Awareness

PHASES OF CYCLIC MEDITATION:

Increased intensity

Maximal intensity

Decreased intensity

Minimal intensity

TECHNIQUE:

1. Lie down in shavasana. -legs apart,Hands by the side of the body and palms facing upwards, fingers semiflexed,eyes closed.

Keep your face relaxed with a gentle smile on your face.

2. "PRAYER"chant the shloka.

3. Perform Instant Relaxation technique(IRT) for 1 minute.

4. Come to tadasana stithi(Centering).

5. Relaxation and centering in Tadasana.

6. Perform Ardhakatichakrasana.

7. To perform Ardhakatichakrasana, come down to your right side with right arm fully stretched and left palm on left thigh.This is known as Linear awareness.

8. Perform Shavasana and feel the surface awareness.

9.Perform Quick Relaxation Technique(QRT) for 3 minutes.

10. After that come to Dandasana(Come up and relax in leg stretched forward and back sti and erect posture)

11. Perform Vajrasana(By bending your knees backward and sitting on the heels)

12.Next perform Shashankasana(By bending forward from

Vajrasana and your head touchinh the ground and palms place forward on the ground and come back to vajrasana again.

10. Perform Ushtrasana(By coming up from vajrasana and bending backward and try to catch hold of your heels at the back)

11. Release in leg stretched position(Dandasana)

12.Then go back to shavasana

13. Perform Deep Relaxation Technique(DRT) for 14 minutes.

14. Come up straight or with support to Vajrasana.

15.End with Shanthi mantra or by chanting three rounds of omkara.

PRACTICE NOTE:

1. Eyes should be closed throughout the practice.
2. Focus and listen to instruction and follow them.
3. Preferably practice in evening after work or daily routine.
4. Slow and continous steady movements should be there during the performance of yogic postures. Perfection of asanas

never means to say that one has attained the focus of mind. It is the way you perform the entire cyclic meditation without any

disturbances defines your awareness.

What do you get by the practice of Cyclic Meditation?

The series of stimulation involved in cyclic meditation helps to relax the body and also solve the major complexities of mind.In one of the research article I have come across, it suggests that practise of Cyclic meditation is known to reduce occupational stress in particular. It is also known to reduce heart rate by bringing about sympathovagal balance and also vagal dominance as such and maintenance of good cardiac health.A strong sympathovagal balance ensures stable cardiovascular function as cardiovascular system is primarily under the control of Autonomic nervous system. There was also increased breath volume and decreased oxygen consumption as suggested in the research article of Dr Sherley telles thus helping to decrease excessive body's energy expenditure. As the prayer of Cyclic mediation tells we are always in between the two extreme states of being agitated or being inactive. So the basic idea behind Cyclic meditation is to achieve the state of equilibrium by combining 'awakening' and 'calming'down practices. The period of practicing yogic postures constitutes the 'awakening' aspects while periods of supine rest constitutes 'calming' practices and thus helping us to achieve a perfect state of equilibrium.Try to find yourself a yoga guru and get going with this aspect of Cyclic meditation in your upcoming days!!

PRANIC ENERGISATION TECHNIQUE(PET)

Pranic Energisation Technique is a technique developed by Svyasa which aims at energising each and every system and organ of our body by using pranic shakti. It involves Pranamaya kosha and forms a part of Integrated Approach of

Yogic Therapy. Breathing is the outward manifestation of prana."Breath" is the bridge between mind & body, so by exercising proper breathing techniques one gets mastery over the mind and leads to joyful and peaceful state for the divine pursuits.

Now let's move on to the technique of PET as such:

TECHNIQUE:

Prayer:

Pranasyedam Vashe sarvam tridiveyat Pratishtitham

maateva putran rakshasva sreescha pragnamcha videhina iti.

Whatever exists in three worlds, it is all under the control of Prana. Prana protects us as a mother protects her child. Prana

gives us affluence and intelligence. "Breathing" is the outward manifestation of "Prana".

1. Recognition of Breath imbalances:

-Feel the breath at the tip of your nose.

-Relax all the parts of your body

-Feel the air going in and out of your nostrils(Watch the breath)as the inhalation becomes continous, slow and rhythmic so as the

exhalation. Recognoise the breath going inside the nose,throat,bronchiles and lungs and recognoise the

breath coming up from lungs,throat and nose.

-Now recognoise the imbalance between the two nostrils where one nostril is more free than the other.

-Slowly the imbalance reduces as the air goes in and out.

2. Nadishuddhi pranayama -If imbalance still present perform Nadishuddhi pranayama for 9 rounds.

3. Extend the awareness from the tip of the nose to the lungs.

4. Practice 9 rounds of inhalation and exhalation.

-Observe the cool air coming inside and warm air going outside.

5.Recognoise the vyana

-Adopt chin mudra and place it on thigh.

-Feel the sensation of nerve impulses passing to brain from the arms.

-Feel the Heart beat.

-Now release the ngers and again bring contact of the two fingers in chin mudra.

-Trace the nerve impulse.

-Practise this for 9 rounds.

-Then practise chinmaya(practises by folding all the three ngers in chin mudra except thumb and index nger) and aadi

mudra(by folding the thumb and closing the remaining fingers over the thumb)

-Then practise Namaskara mudra by bringing both the palms
together and feel the heart beat and pulse.Feel the palms.
-Nerve impulse slowly moving from palms to brain. Slowly press both the palms. Chant 'M' kara and feel the resonance.
-Now slowly seperate the palms and move them away from each other and then join them again.
-Continue this movement for few rounds and feel the space between palms getting sensitized.
Experience vyana in that space.
-Now rotate the palms clockwise and anticlockwise churning the vyana.Repeat this for few rounds.
6.Movement and rotation of Vyana:
-Now place the palms on the knees and start moving the prana(vyana) from the right heel, calf muscle,from under the thigh, right buttock, right lower back and all along the way upto the shoulder.Then move the prana from the fingers, to the wrist, forearms,upper arm, shoulder and join this prana at the shoulder level below the neck along the prana which was brought from below the heels. Then move it upwards from the back of the head and coming down to the right forehead, right eye, right nostril down to the right side of the neck, chest and abdomen,further down to the right pelvis,thigh, knees and shin right upto the toes. Also move the vyana downwards from the shoulders upto the fingers.Repeat the same on left side and then both sides.
8)Balancing and energisation of Vyana:
-We shall now move the vyana from the higher density region to the lower density region. For this we have to always compare the energy densities on different sides of

the body. Observe the imbalance of energies by comparing right side of the body with the left side and then front side with the back side.After recognising then try to balance by allowing the flow of prana from higher density to lower density region. After this practice vyana gets balanced and one feels relaxed and calm within.

1. Silence: Feel the prana around the body which is expanding and diusing the cosmic universe.

Experience the blissful state of silence.

Try to remain in this state for as long as possible.

2. Resolve: Take a resolution and repeat it for 9-10 times within.

3. Ending the practice: End the practice slowly by chanting shanti mantra or 3

rounds of omkara for the well being of the entire universe.

MIND SOUND RESONANCE TECHNIQUE(MSRT)

Pranic energisation technique has been found to be very much beneficial in healing when focussed for particular tissues during

the balancing of vyana(step 8) by increasing the flow to that injured tissue and thus promote healing. It has also been found to be good relieving deep rooted emotions.Now all you have to do is just find a yoga guru and start practising it under the guidance of him!!

Let's go on with our next technique that is Mind Sound Resonance technique. It is an advanced technique which can take you to the deeply rested state of mind body complex by bringing about resonance all over your body. Before going on with the technique as such let us try to understand the three

words Mind, Sound and Resonance.

What is Mind?

Each one of us percieve mind in our own different ways and give our own explanations about it. Some people will make very much effective utilisation of their minds whereas others keep it safely in their lockers making it to perish.According to many of the hardcore neuroscientists, mind

is the expression of activity of brain cells known as

neurons.According to psychologists it's the sum total of the cognitive functions carried out by a wakeful mind. But Yoga defines mind as a conglomeration of thoughts. So many different thoughts are grouped together and reside in mind. These thoughts which

arise and grouped in our mind are of two types:

1. Manifest mind and
2. Unmanifest mind.

Manifest mind is cognizable as in wakeful and dream states whereas the unmanifest mind is dormant as in

deep sleep state. Our thinking apparatus is the Mind which is responsible for both Manomaya kosha and Vijnanamaya kosha.

Mind in manomaya kosha is said to percieve and understand the inputs from the senses and play the emotions also called Bhavana. These emotions are so much powerful that they can alter the electrical and physiological activity of brain. These negative emotions which are six in number as follows:1) Kama(Intense desire) 2)Krodha(Anger) 3)Lobha(greed) 4)Moha(Infatuation) 5)Mada(Arrogance) and 6)Matsarya(Jealousy) which are

also known as Purusharthas which are supressed and stored in subconscious mind percolates the physical body and lead to

chronic imbalances in our body.So one's duty is to be free from all these emotions.

What is Sound?

Sound according to science is a form of energy which requires a medium to travel. Human ear can percieve sound ranging from 20-2000Hz frequency. In Yoga, we define sound as Sabda.This sound is much broader and intense than the sound percieved in Science. Sabda is

Spanda i.e., a wave. It is of two types:1) audible(ahata) and 2) inaudible(anahata). In one of our lecture we were taught that sound as the quality of akasha. "Sabdhagunanam akasam", defining yoga as taking the quality of akasha. Anahata is the unheard sound or the mental sound.Whatever the internal dialogue takes place though the thoughts which are nothing but words known as Anahata shabda which is said to represent the entire universe. Yogis hear this sound by the intense practice of Brahmari pranayama or any other forms of meditation.

What is Resonance?

As we all have studied in science, when the frequency of any object or any functional system matches with its natural frequency then the object or the functional system vibrates with the maximal amplitude. This is known as Resonance.This has been used in variety of aspects in our daily lives as in case of tuning of musical instruments. This same phenonenon has been used in MSRT.

What is Silence?

Silence is a state where there is no thoughts or a state where you are not aware of them. Swami Ramakrishna paramahamsa defines it with an example. A salt doll wanted to measure the depth of the ocean. What happened when it plunged into the ocean? It dissolved itself in the ocean retaining no individuality whatsoever and became one with the ocean.

The state of pure silence as such is a state wherein you dissolve yourself in the oneness of existence.

What is Resolve?

A clearly thought out, well formulated positive thought with minimum words forms resolution or sankalpa. The resolution whatever one takes should be for the sake of others and it should not be with a purpose to harm others physically, mentally or spiritually.Thus we repeat the resolution nine times at the end of practice to reach the inner pure state of silence.. After knowing the basic concepts of MSRT as

such let's move onto it's technique.

TECHNIQUE:

1)OPENING PRAYER:

Mahamrutyunjaya mantra:

Om trayambakam yajamahe
sugandhim pushtivardhanam
urvarukamiurvarukamiva bandhanat
mryutyormukshi yamamrutat
Om santi santi santih.

We offer our salutation to the three eyed Lord Shiva for increasing vitality, fragrance in us, release us from the bondage of

death, just like a ripened cucumber fully.

1. First stage:Ahatha chanting of A,U, M and AUM and feel resonance.

3)Second stage: -Chanting 'A'kara -Ahatha-Anahatha for 5 rounds.

-Chanting 'U'kara-Ahatha-Anahatha for 5 rounds

-Chanting 'M'kara-Ahatha-Anahatha for 5 rounds.

-Chanting 'U'kara-Ahatha-Anahatha for 5 rounds.

-Chanting 'AUM' kara-Ahatha-Anahatha for 5 rounds.

-Feel the resonance mentally.

Ahata:Mahamrutyunjaya mantra

Feel the resonance

Ahatha-Anahatha-Mahamrutyunjaya mantra.

-Feel the resonance.

4) Anahatha chanting of AUM

Feel the resonance

5) Ajapajapa 'AUM' to silence and feel the resonance of OM coming up and spreading throughout the body and diffusing into

silence.

6) Stay in silence.

7) Resolve

8) Shanti mantra or end the practice by chanting 3 rounds of OM kara.

This is one such wonderful technique to eradicate our unwanted negative thoughts and achieve the state of equilibrium

or attain samattvam. Therefore let's go on with the practice of MSRT in our upcoming days!!

MASTERING THE EMOTIONS TECHNIQUE(MEMT)

Emotions are very important and a way for expressing our inner feelings. There is no living being in this srishti or creation which is there without emotion. A man without emotions can also never be said as a healthy being. Whether positive or negative a man is composed of emotions. Emotions play a central role in the evolution of consciousness and influence the emergence of higher levels of awareness during ontogeny,We should never supress our emotion but instead try to master them. Once we start mastering our emotions we tend to even welcome the negative emotions and this provides another opportunity to know about ourseleves.Opening the emotional gates within us leads to the discovery of truth within us. It is often said, "Jump into the river of emotion that will take you the ocean of truth".Many of us in today's society are suffering from supressed emotions and MEMT is one such technique that helps in cleansing the supressed emotions.If your emotions are supressed your full creative potential is not released.Learn

to release the supressed emotions completely for effective learning and to induce creativity at its full potential is the concept of MEMT.

TECHNIQUE:

Opening prayer:
"Yallabdhva Puman Siddho Bhavati Amrtho Bhavati Tripto Bhavati"
Prayer taken from the Narada bhakthi sutras explains as such by attaining the stage of transcedental devotional service in pure love of god, one becomes perfect, immortal and peaceful.

1.Recognoise thinking vs feeling: Try to observe what is there in your mind from the third person's point of view. Feel and observe yourself and see how your feelings are. Do not suppress the thoughts. As it is done for longer time, thoughts gets weaker.
Now take a deep breath and let everything go. Feel free, light and relax completely.
2. Art of Sublimation: Slow down the breathing and speed of your thoughts. Sublimation is the art of slowing down your reactions. Breathing is calm, Body is stable and light. Let go of the thoughts and try to relax.
3. Invoke-Intensify-Diuse: Invoke by starting to listen soft bhajans or namavalis. Enjoy and merge in the rhythm of the music and bhava of surrenderance to the God. Amplify the emotion as the speed of the bhajan increases and raga goes on to the higher octave. Let go and allow yourself to get lost in the joy of
the speeded up loop of repitition of God's name. Intensify further as the speed of namavali increases and feel the vibrations
all over the body. Now diffuse. Continue to listen but stop singing and experience the sound vibrations still resonating in your whole body. Listen to the music diffusing into the space around,the sky and the infinity. Stay on this mood as

the singing stops.

3. Pairs of Opposites: a) Heat and Cold

b) Stretch and relax

c)Constrict and expand

d) Sukha(Happiness) and dukha(Sorrow)

e) Mana(Respect/Honour) and Apamana(Insult)

f) Punya(Virtue) and Apunya(Vice)

In this stage of pairs of opposites, you will recall two extreme opposite experiences from your past. After this step let go of all the emotions that you have recalled and feel free. Recognoise your place or position and feel free that you are here and now everything has gone. Feel the silence.

1. Actions towards different emotions:

• Here at first we have to recall our experiences of developing friendliness towards a happy person,"Maitri".Let go of this experience. Relax completely.

-Now, visualize yourself showing compassion to someone who is suffering. Drop this experience and let go and relax.

-Next imagine yourself of being "Mudita" i.e., being delighted and feel glad towards a person who is always helpful and useful

to others.Let go and relax.

-Lastly, recall or imagine a situation that you show indifference to a wicked, cruel and harmful person,"Upeksha".Let go and be free from everything.

-Visualise moving from one experience to other, Inhale deeply and exhale completely. Let go and completely diffuse.

1. Death Experience:

-Slowly go back and lie down in shavasana.

-Collapse the whole body on the oor.

-You are going to experience Physical death.

-Your breathing is slowing down and has almost stopped.

-Thoughts slow down and organs cease to function one by one.

-Mind subside in silence.

-Now you just experienced death of ego, and that physical death is not real death.

-Become aware of your own body and breath slowly and come to sitting position.

2. Silence:

-Happiness is Silence,Bliss is Silence, Silence leads to Pure consciousness.

-Now feel the silence and bliss,the innite silence like the innite blue sky. Diuse into expansive awareness of silence. Stay as

long as you can. If thoughts come up, feel the wave of resonance and all the waves diuse into silence.

3. Resolve: From that blissful state of silence arises a positive thought in the form of a positive resolution which is a short

statement with a minimum number of words. Repeat preferably in your mother tongue in present continous tense for

atleast 10 times and allow it to diffuse on the bed of silence.

Closing Prayer: Chant Shanti Mantra or 3 rounds of Omkara for the well being of entire universe and end the practice.

The biggest emotion that is said to be the cause of all the suffering and distress is Love.Be it child or an adolecent or adult

or old age, when one doesn't get this, it will result in distress.Insufficient nurture from mother(as a baby) or insucient
friendship(sharing and caring) as an adolescent, or insufficient opportunity to enjoy the parenthood(only giving) and not receiving the same love from children, are all said to be the causes of distress. Understanding and recognosing these emotions introspectively and growing into the expectation real
parenthood without expectation is a technique to gain emotional stability.The next aspect to be kept in mind is the thing
called "Universal love" as said earlier wherein the joy of giving is not restricted to your offspring or to your loved ones but to the
entire universe.You become a one with the Universe. It doesn't happen by itself. It requires our strict Sadhana with specific
practices like MEMT under the guidance of a spiritual master. So let's start to nurture our positive emotions by develop positive
thoughts and love for others to be healthy and joyful!!

MIND IMAGERY TECHNIQUE(MIRT)

Mind Imagery Technique is one among the Integrated Approaches of Yoga Therapy to strengthen the Immune defense for combating cancer and other disorders. MIRT is said to work at the Manomaya kosha level.Mind Imagery technique the capacity of our mind to use visual power in the form of imageries.While the MSRT focuses on the ability of mind to experience the sound MIRT uses the visual aspect ofmind and thus provide relaxation and happiness. The visuals or imageries are of two types as such:

1. Active and 2. Neutral visuals.

Active visuals are those in which we get lost. These are the images which we do not have control because of their speed and packing energy which are

further of two types:

1. Positive and 2. Negative visuals. Positive images are those powerful imageries which are the joyful moments in our life

which trigger positiveness within oneself while the negative ones are those which trigger violent emotions such anger, fear,

tension, anxiety, etc.,and which bind us our samskaras. Neutral imageries are those which are under our control

and they come
and go and their energy and awareness is maintained in body.
Coming to the technique of MIRT as such,it is as follows.
TECHNIQUE:
3. PRAYER
Anekabahudara vaktnanetram Pasyami tvam sarvato
nantarupam Nantam na madhyam na punastavadim
Pasyami visvesvara visvarupa
- Bhagavadgita
"Many hands, abdomen, faces and eyes, I see you.O Lord Krishna, spread everywhere to infinite dimensions. Neither do I see the
beginning, middle or the end. This is the Universal Vision I see.
As earlierly said this whole creation is a maya as such and still it's completely unexplained. An instance of this maya was the
Krishna preaching Bhagavadgita to Arjuna amid the battlefield.
How could he do that? Where did he get time? Many say all that knowledge of Bhagavadgita came to Arjuna from Krishna by the
divine Vision of Vishvarupa. For this even Arjuna was given special vision when he was unable to see that Viratadarshana of the
Lord.That was the power of Universal Vision. Hence we have to close our eyes and recall this wonderful vision of unending form
of the Lord as explained in the shloka.
1. Recognise Active and Passive(Neutral) imageries:
-Lie down comfortably in shavasana.

-In a passive way, as a witness, observe the thoughts in the form of visuals on your mental screen.
-Observe the thoughts. So many thoughts come and go. In some of the thoughts you realise that you are actively plunged into it
by losing awareness. Continue the practice. For some thoughts you realise that they come and go but your awareness is kept
up. Those thoughts for which your awareness was retained are the neutral thoughts and for those for which your awareness
was lost are the Active thoughts. Further observe whether the Active thoughts you were involved with were positive or negative.Positive thoughts induce growth and creativeness whereas the negative thoughts like fear and anger cause destruction.
3)Shift between Active and Passive imageries(Contract-Expand) : Here we deal with two aspects, one is focussing and the other is defocussing. Focussing is done by the practice of Dharana such as trataka whereas defocussing is done by the practice of Dhyana. Thus we tend to shift the imagery from its passive
or neutral state to active state by Dharana and then try to shift this back to active state by Dhyana and vice versa. We tend to
contract the image by focussing and again tend to expand it by defocussing and so on. This can be practised for 9 rounds by visualising the picture of "OM" also referred as "Visvarupa".
1. Time Dimension(Speed up-Slow down): Here we deal with the increasing and decreasing the frequency of ickering of images. Here we continue to open the eyes and

then see the image of OM or visvarupa. Then we close our eyes and try to visualise
it. After the image disappears then we again open our eyes and see the image of OM and close eyes and visualise until the picture disappears.We continue this process by increasing the speed.Speeding up like this makes the thought active and thus
we try to increase the speed of mind. Now by increasing the speed we are transforming the thought or emotion from passive
to active. The process is dharana.We practice this for 9 rounds.After this we slow down the thought and thus make it passive
again by the process of dhyana. After holding on to the frequency of ickering of image we allow it slow down and almost
still. Thus we feel the relaxation.

2. Mind Imagery: Here we choose an image that we like that helps in strengthening our immune system. The images recommended are ista devatas(personal God), inner sun(bright sun in your heart center) and yantra(like chakras in our pranic body)

Practice step 3 and step 4 for 9 rounds each.

3. Silence: Allow the mind to stay in an expansive blissful state of silence(Visualise an infinite sky and merge into it). Observe
the continous ow of awareness with no thoughts in your mind.

4. Resolve: Take any sankalpa or resolution and repeat it for 9 rounds. The sankalpa you take should never be negative or
harmful to the society but it should be positive and

constructive in nature.

5. Ending the Practice: End the practice by chanting shanti mantra or by chanting 3 rounds of omkara for the well being of
the entire universe.

After knowing so much about the Mind Imagery technique let's try out this wonderful technique under the guidance of a yogic
master and experience the Universal vision within us!!

VIJNANA SADHANA KAUSALAM(VISAK)

Let us move on to another technique which is also a part of Integrated aprroaches of Yoga therapy known as Vijana Sadhana Kausalam. It is aimed at strengthening Vijnanamaya kosha and has been developed by Svyasa. VISAK is a technique which works on fear. Fear has been always there in every man right from his childhood.According to yoga it begins in the manomaya kosha and due to the dominating emotions one gets into the likes and dislikes resulting in the blockage of prana resulting in vyadhi at the annamaya level. In vijnanamaya kosha it results in individualisation or ego. The solution to overcome fear is by the analysis and interpretation of ourselves during fearful situations to get a proper solution.Fear sometimes can be good as it triggers the flight or fight response within us during stressful situation. But sometimes sustained fear deep within us can lead to problems and ill health and affect our sadhana.So here as said earlier recognition and analysis forms the major aspect which has been dealt with in VISAK. Now let's move on to the technique as such!!

TECHNIQUE:

1. Prayer:

-Make yourself comfortable in any meditative posture with

hands in chin mudra.
-Keep your back and neck erect and your eyes closed and slowly chant the prayer.
Dikkaladyanavacchinna
nantachinamtramurthaye
Svanubhutayekamanaya namah Shantaya tejase
Yogavasishta
Salutations to that innite intelligence beyond space and time which is pure consciousness and peace embodied and which can
be measured only be Self-realisation.
1. Happiness analysis: Recall an incidence of greatest happiness in your life. Relive that happiness. Many of our holy
scriptures always tells us that happiness is not found in material objects. True happiness always comes from within, from the
inner state of silence.Inner silence is bliss and bliss is happiness. We all have to tune to our
innite silence, the core of our inner being.
2. FEAR ANALYSIS: -Recall an incident that invoked
fear. Observe the experience of the fear as an observer.
-Examine whether it is fear of illness, death of relatives, fear of losing fame and so on.
-How does fear make one feel?
Positive, focussed,limited,constricted, etc., Now how to overcome the fear? The answer is by properly training up the
body to face the fear.And keep the mind calm.
-Fear is always present within us and it's been in a natural more precisely has become a 'survival instinct' within us. Fear has got

two got two components with it:

1) fear at physical level and

2)fear of mental level.

• Fear at physical level are the ones such as disease and death.

• Fear at mental level are those such as fear of losing job, fear of insult and so on.

• And because of the overactivity of our senses even the physical fear has also been a part of psychological or mental fear as such.

• As said in one of my chapters the major fear within us is the fear of death. Non acceptance of this event of our life has been the cause leading to absence of life within us even though we are alive.

• Be ready to accept the death even though it banging the door at your next moment of life.

• Fear itself is never a contradictive as such, it can become harmful only when we start running away from it. Overcome it by facing it and acceptance of the reality. When we start to face it with courage it becomes a thrill as it happens in the case if sky diving and when watching horror movies. Fear is movement of mind and happiness is silence of mind. The solution to fear is proper understanding.

1. Fear-Happiness combine: -Invoke fear. Observe the changes in all levels-physical, mental,emotional,intellectual and spiritual.

-Analyse the fear, diuse and normalise.

-Expand the fear to fearlessness, and from fearlessness to

blissful state through right understanding.

-Realisation of our true nature and proper analysis and introspection for the reason of fear is necessary.

-Completely relax.

2. Sreyas-Preyas combine:

-To overcome fear and be fearless observe the your lifestyle.

-Start observing how you are? How is your diet, action towards others?Are you active, lazy or exaggerated?

-Start observing the guna which is dominant in you(Sattva-active, tamo-lazy,dormant or rajasic-Exaggerated).

-Completely overcome fear by moving from the state of preyas to sreyas.Preyas is selfishness and Sreyas is selflessness.

-Controlling ourselves for a reason of liking or enjoying something for a higher good to come in future is known as preyas whereas on the contrary going with our likes or enjoyment even though we know we should avoid those is known as

sreyas. A person in this state can never overcome fear and is always said to experience the lower state of bliss or the one which

is temporary. Therefore one should never mistake it for the real bliss for the real bliss always lies beyond our senses. Remember

selflessness and fearless are the only means to achieve the real bliss. Fear is movement whereas silence is bliss.

-If one has to experience this blissful and fearless state, one has to let go whatever that comes through senses and practice complete detachment or vairagya. This is the only way to overcome fear and achieve selflessness.

3. Silence:

-Now feel the silence and bliss, the infinite silence like the infinite blue sky. Dffiuse into expansive awareness of silence. Stay as long as you can. If thoughts come up, feel the wave of resonance and all the waves diffuse into silence.

-Try to move from the fearful state to the fearless state.

-Always remember at this state of silence you will find solutions to many of your problems.Whatever the problems that you used to consider as complicated are generated with solutions automatically in this ultimate blissful state of silence.Hence one must resort to silence for sometime atleast once in a day preferably early morning.

4. Resolve:

-From that blissful state of silence arises a positive thought in the form of a positive resolution which is a short statement with a minimum number of words. Repeat preferably in your mother tongue in present continous tense for atleast 10 times and allow it to diffuse on the bed of silence.

5. Closing prayer:

• Chant Shanti Mantra or 3 rounds of Omkara for the well being of entire universe and end the practice.

So let's get going with the practice of VISAK technique and be fearless and be the leaders of tomorrow!!

ANANDA AMRTA SINCHANA(ANAMS)

Ananda Amrta Sinchana is one of the advanced techniques which is also a part of Integrated Approaches ofYoga Therapy. The word Ananda means 'bliss', amrta is 'nectar' and sinchana is 'sprinkling'. It means" Sprinkling the blissful depth from your inner nature which is your true self. It operates on the Annamaya kosha and has its origin from taittareya upanishad and has been developed by svyasa.

Happiness analysis: In this today's world we all have been wandering for happiness. We all are in the misconception that happiness is derived from the external world but never know that we ourselves possess happiness within. The whole creation is from bliss that resides within us. All beings are born out of

bliss. They sustain in bliss and finally merge into bliss. I alwaysthink about how luxury has been mistaken for happiness in our society. But luxury never gives happiness as such, even if at all if you believe you may get it, the happiness derived is only momentary. Just imagine a 5 chocolates with you and four friends

around you. You may get happiness by eating all the chocolate but that's only momentary. Just try to eat all the chocolates in front of them without sharing. I bet you

cannot have it with complete heart and you never enjoy it's taste or flavour as such though you may show so much happiness outside while having them. This is luxury, though it may seem like happiness its never the same inside. Now let's share the chocolate with all your friends and eat it. You will surely be happy from within and out. This is true happiness or bliss. Sharing and caring others also forms an important aspect of true happiness. Now
let's move on to the technique of ANAMS.

TECHNIQUE:

1. PRAYER:

-Make yourself comfortable in any meditative posture with hands in chin mudra.

-Keep your back and neck erect and your eyes closed and slowly chant the prayer.

Anando brahmeti vyajanat
Anandadhyeva kalvimani bhutani jayante Anandaa
prayantya abhiabhisaavichanteti Sa parame vyoman pratinohita

-Taittareya upanishad

2. Recall the blissful Silence:

-Observe complete silence for sometime.

-Try to recall the happy moments and joyful experiences of your life.

-You can't search for happiness from anywhere nor you can buy it for money in this world.

-True happiness is always there within you. To discover that,one needs to search within.As they say "To get something you need to lose something". "To get true happiness, you need to lose your ego and greed".

-Always try to be compassionate to the society around you for it acts as key to open the lock of true happiness within

you.
-Remember bliss is silence and silence is always pure consciousness. If consciousness is the base of creation then bliss is the the
energy at the base of this physical universe.
3. Bliss in Pairs of Opposites:
-Next we will go on enjoying the bliss with the pair of opposites by adopting shavasana.
• Recall and experience where you are walking through an extremely hot environment like a desert. You are sweat, thirsty
and also exhausted.Your feets are burning and and you feel like collapsing.Be in that condition and feel the heat.Recognoise
the bliss in that condition.Now the question is how to experience the bliss in that state? The answer lies in yoga itself as it
says-"yogasthah kuru karmani"-accomplish this by being established in yoga state-the ocean of bliss-the silence. The state
of yoga here is going through that hot condition. Whenever you face any situation by adopting it, you never feel the worst
part of it. Instead you start getting out the essence of happiness and joy that lies deep within that circumstance. -Now drop
this, and recall yourself being in an experience of extreme cold condition like being in antartica.In a snowy,windy day you are
wearing extremely thin clothes and shivering. Your hands and feet are numb and you feel like running away from the place.But in the background you are enjoying the inner

state of bliss or essence of happiness of that situation by completely
adopting to it.You may have heard about soldiers living in extremely terrible conditions? How do they do that? Its just by
training their body and mind to adopt to that situation and yoga does the same thing.That is the reason why nowadays Yoga and breathing exercises are being taught to so many soldiers who work at higher altitudes to help for their survival by
adopting to those situations.

• Next move to experience a situation of being clean like moving in a beautiful garden which is very well taken care of. Enjoy
bliss in this beautiful garden with so much beautiful flowers and birds around. Now shift your experience of being in a dirty
place. Imagine that place full of dirt and trash everywhere with flies around and stinking. Recall and relive that experience. But
in the background part you are enjoying the bliss even in that situation by completely adopting it.

-Next let's move on to a situation of being in a complete bright area.You can imagine a place where it's so bright that you are unable to open your eyes.

Recognoise bliss in light. Now shift your mind to the opposite experience of being in completely dark. You are unable to see
anything. Recognoise bliss in darkness. After this,let go off all the memories and just relax.

4.Ananda in both Action and Non-Action: We are always in a state of action.Running around in our lives to fulfill our needs and also in search of comfort and happiness but what matters is how happy are we in doing that! We need to evaluate this by finding out happiness in between our state of action and non-action for there lies the real happiness. When the mind is kept active all the time nor if it kept dormant as in the case of deep sleep we can never find the source of happiness. To find out the source of happiness one must go to a state that is in between these two i.e., the state of silence. Silence is bliss and from this blissful state of silence one has to extend this Ananda during the state of action and non-action.

5. Love all: In our today's society "Love" has been always seen and felt as a relationship between persons.But love is more beyond that than being physical.Love is always an unconditioned aspect wherein we learn to give without expecting anything in return.People consider to show love, one should be attached,its never like that you can practice love without being attached called as anabhisnehah by Sri krishna. That is the way to avoid attachments in your life and there arises the real bliss.

Instead of being posessive about person or an event you learn to give your part in sharing and caring for the world around.If you want happiness you should never stick on to loving the comforted ones but serve the suering ones by showing your love towards them Love all and hate none. Love even the ones who brought down you in lives. There reduces all

your
negative emotions and you can find the essence of happiness within.Hence start spreading unattached love everywhere
with knowledge and understanding.

1. Spread Ananda everywhere: -As they say whatever kept stored within you for a long time spoils. Whether it is wealth,food or anything as such. It should always be shared. So start spreading the happiness all around. Learn to make everyone
happy around.Let everyone be happy and blissful because that is the one that retains your happiness for a long time.As a poet
says,"If the whole world is happy and you are sad. The world can make you be happy. But if the whole world is sad and you alone
want to experience happiness it is never possible".Hence find the joy in serving others and loving everyone and everything around you.
2. Resolve: From the depth of silence, try taking a positive thought about spreading happiness all around and serving the
community around. Feel the happiness around and within you.Now let go, relax completely and prepare yourself for ending the practice with closing prayer.
3. Closing prayer: Chant Shanti Mantra or 3 rounds of Omkara for the well being of entire universe and end the practice.

Our Mind or Chit is always occupied with worldly things which are temporary that never gives permanent happiness. Then the
Chit is called Asat (untrue) or Ashuddha (impure) Chit. It

is only when the Chit is occupied with the Self, the pure soul within,

which is Eternal, there is an experience of permanent happiness and Bliss (Anand). That is the only Sat (Satya - Truth), and that's

when the Chit is called Sat Chit or Shuddha (pure) Chit which is experienced complete silence within us.So let's get get going

and practice this wonderful technique under the guidance of a yogic guru and make our lives blissful!!

THE FIVE VAYUS

Through the severe meditative poses and breath regulations, the Yogis discovered that Prana or the Life energy as such could be divided into subunits or energy components called as Vayus(Winds). The Five Vayus have specific function and particular direction of flow as such. Through the
conscious control of this prana Vayus they were not only able to maintain optimal health but also were able to activate the
Kundalini energy dormant at the base of the spine. Coming to the Vayus as such, "Vayu" in sanskrit means "wind" And va as
such means "one which flows".So by this we understand that the basic function of the Vayu is to ow throughout the body and
thus regulate the body functions. The ancient yogis found 49 distinct types of Vayus out of which 5 have been considered as
signicant named as " Pancha Vayus".These five primary energy currents are as such:

1.Prana-Vayu
2.Apana-Vayu
3.Samana-Vayu
4.Udana-Vayu
5.Vyana-Vayu

Let's understand about each Vayu as such:

1.Prana-Vayu: Prana-Vayu is situated in the heart and it's energy pervades the chest region. It translates as "forward moving air"

and it flows inwards and upwards. It governs the reception of food, air, senses and thought and represents element air.Its expression is said to be cyclical and also said to feed or nourish the other vayus. To strengthen the prana Vayu Heart opening poses like Bridge pose, Camel pose, Cobra pose and pranayamas like Nadishodana, Brahmari can be practiced.

2.Apana-Vayu: Apana Vayu is situated in the pelvic floor and it's energy pervades the lower abdomen. It is translated as "the air that moves away," and its flow is downwards and out. Its energy nourishes the organs of digestion, reproduction, and elimination.If it's action is elimination, it represents steadiness

and element earth.If Apana Vayu is disturbed one starts to feel weakness in legs. Hence to strengthen Apana vayu one must

start practising releasing poses like forward bending asanas and seated twists. Practicing kriyas such as nauli, agnisara will also

do the job.

3.Samana-Vayu: Samana-Vayu is situated in the abdomen with its energy centered in the navel. Samana-Vayu translates to "the

balancing air" and its flow moves from the periphery of the body to the center. It governs the digestion and assimilation of

all substances: food, air, experiences, emotions, and

thoughts.This Vayu's action is assimilation, its expression is internal, and its associated chakras

dence and a lack of motivation and desire. Issues with digestion can be related to disturbed SamanaVayu. To strengthen the Samana vayu focus your asana practice on twisting poses and core-strengthening yoga poses. Practice Kapalabhati Pranayama with Uddiyana Bandha and Agni Sara

Kriya. Bringing awareness of Samana-Vayu in any yoga pose creates a focus to open and release the digestive fire and its elements are Manipura and fire. A weak or dysfunctional Samana-Vayu can manifest as poor judgment, low concentration and indigestion in the body.

4.Udana-Vayu: Udana-Vayu is situated in the throat and it has a circular flow around the neck and head. Udana-Vayu translates

to "that which carries upward," and its ow moves upward from the heart to the head, five senses, and brain. It functions to

"hold us up" and governs speech, self-expression, and growth.This Vayu's action is metabolization, its expression is verbal, and its associated chakras and elements are Vishuddha & Ajna and ether. A weak or dysfunctional Udana-Vayu can manifest as speech diculties, shortness of breath and diseases of the

throat. A lack of self-expression, uncoordinated movement or loss of balance can be related to disturbed Udana-Vayu. To strengthen Udana-Vayu practice Ujjayi Pranayama and

Bhramari Pranayama with Jalandhara Bandha. Focus on practicing inversions and backbending yoga poses that bring energy to the neck, shoulders, and head.Awareness on Udana vayu helps to maintain a long spine and increases focus toward the practice.

5.Vyana-Vayu: Vyana-Vayu is situated in the heart and lungs and flows throughout the entire body. Vyana-Vayu translates

as "outward moving air," and its ow moves from the center of the body to the periphery. It governs the circulation of all substances throughout the body and assists the other Vayus with their functions. This Vayu's action is circulation, its expression is alignment, and its associated chakras and elements are Svadisthana and water. A weak or dysfunctional VyanaVayu can create feelings of separation and alienation and can create disjointed, fluctuating and rambling thoughts. Poor circulation, impaired nerve stimulation, skin disorders, and nervous breakdowns can be related to disturbed Vyana-Vayu.

Practice pranayama with kumbhaka (breath retention). Focus your asana practice more on vinyasa movements like the Sun

Salutations to circulate prana and blood. Bringing awareness of Vyana-Vayu in any yoga pose creates a focus on strength and fluid movement of the body.

Apart from these Pancha pranas there are "Upapranas" which are five in number that regulate various actions. They are as follows:

1. Naga is the air which regulates burping.
2. Kurma is the one which regulates contracting movements like blinking of eyes.
3. Krikala is the upaprana that governs sneezing.

4. Devadatta controls yawning.
5. Dhananjaya controls functioning of heart valves. Having known all these one must strict resort to the practice of pranayama to control the flow of these currents in the body so as to enhance the vitality of body and mind.

THE MYSTERY OF DEATH

"Death" is one word we all know is somewhat unexplained even today.Every person has his own explanations when asked about death. Some say it as
very much painful, some call it as relief, some people are not even ready to accept death. We all from our childhood days have been learnt that death is somewhat frightening. But have we ever wondered why death itself is so much frightening?
Maybe each one of us has their own theory to debate upon for that. Now before moving further let us know the reason for our fear about death.Let me explain you an example to share my view. Now imagine yourself to be asked to walk along a dark path or through a dark forest all alone. How would you feel? Scared right!!Now can you tell me the reason for that. The reason is all simple, the reason is we are not destined or know where we would reach because we have not seen the other end or nobody has told us about the end or destination. The same thing is what has happened for our fear of Death.This is also the reason why people are unable to lead a beautiful lives because of the fear of this unknown theory of death. You may think that people know what happens after death from a theological point of view as written in the Holy books but this is not sufficient in our minds since it lacks actual proof or living evidence. The fear

of death has also been fueled by unsatisfactory lives we all are living. Imagine a condition wherein we are leaving exam Hall without completing all the answers. It doesn't feel good right and we are scared what would happen with our next life right!!

Same thing is what happens with death. We all are engaged with our own responsibilities and also the greed of gaining more and more that we don't want to give an end. Hence with these engaged with these stus and greediness we are scared of the state of uncertainity of death. But should we all consider death as

somewhat ill or unpleasant us the question? No, not at all. Death not as such unpleasant. It is a part of life process. Many a times death can be very much boon. As in case of a bedridden suffering patient with an incurable disease who has unbearable pain all over the day and you go ask him what he wants? He

would say it as liberation. I am not saying that he should die as such, but that is the fact. We all are made, we all act and we all perish one or the other day. The thing is how well we act and end our story is the one that matters. And there are many instincts where people decide their own time of death by comitting suicide. This is a very bad concept or idea that has come up with us nowadays. One must always remember that, Death is an event for which we don't have right over it. Many time I see people particularly youngsters comitting suicide for various reasons.

But remember your life as such has a lot of meaning.You never decided your birth as such and you don't have the right to decide your end. It's always taken care by the Law of nature.One more reason what I feel has made me wonder or somewhat fear about death is the way we are treated after death. We lose our

identity as such. We are never called rahul or ajay as such but referred as "Dead body".And the way they cremate dead bodies whether burning or putting under soil. I always get scared of thinking whether alive or not, how would that body be alone in the graveyard that too in the dark underground where there is

nothing to live upon. But somewhere I was able to come out of this dogma of fear when I was coming across lines by a persian poet Rumi who says, "You need not be afraid of death for you are a deathless soul, and you can't be kept in a dark grave because you are lled with God's glow." One more thing that matters

after death is that we are no longer a part of body now. So who cares what happens with the body? That's what yoga tells us

about speaking body as a temple where soul resides in!! We must always remember that our true identity doesn't come from the

body but it comes from our soul. As I always say every moment of life teach us something and even death. Asking how? Let me explain you about this with a small story. Once there was a young man who was travelling with his master. Suddenly he asked his master, "I fear death. How can I get rid of this fear?" Tell

me," the old man answered, "When you borrow a few coins, are you afraid to give them later back?"

"Of course not," the student answered with surprise, "but what does this have to do with my fear?"

The teacher picked up a small piece of soil from the ground and continued, "You have received your body in

debt with required return. And every bite of bread eaten by you, every sip of water drank by you increases that debt. You are made from
dust on which you walk and the ground is your main creditor, constantly reminding you of this debt. It is pulling you down
towards it. In the end, the ground will swallow you whole, without any remains."
The old man threw the soil into the air, after attaining its fall, he finished, "No matter how high you rise, how long you are in the
ight, you will still need to fall down. That is given. And to cope with the fear of this fall is very easy – stop thinking about yourself as the master of your body. Face the thought that you are just a tenant. And because you don't know the length of your rent, remember that it can end at any second. We are all debtors, and our debts will certainly be recovered, no matter if we are afraid of it or not. So is there a point of being afraid?". So knowing that this we all have to start loving each other as earlier as it is the only means to get rid of this fear. Now for this love we also need not be attached as being attached also raises the fear of death. The fear of leaving alone, sometimes they say being silent and being lonely for a longer time is very dangerous.The danger may be for oneself or for the whole society around as there are either of the chances to get either constructive or destructive thoughts for a person. For all of us we are taught to fear
about death, darkness and graveyard. But it is not so, we all should come out of this.As science says darkness is the way to discover light.Hence death is a part of life cycle and the purpose for which you were locked in your body is

done and you have been set free.The renowned mathematical physicist, Sir Roger Penrose at the University of Oxford and researchers at the Max Planck Institute for Physics in Munich suggest that the physical universe that we live in is only our perception and once our physical bodies die, there is an innite beyond. Some believe that consciousness travels to parallel universes after death.Hence we all should understand that death itself is not a terminal point. The terminal point is to merge our individual cosmic energy that is released during the death of physical body as such with the universal cosmic energy.For that we all should develop the two concepts called Abhyasa and Vairagya as Yoga

says.We all should start serving and loving the people around with a feeling of detachment.The easy way of developing is by

the the sincere practice of yoga. Though I may give you various explanations for you about this form of serving and loving one another with a sense of detachment but the experience of it comes only through the dedicated sadhana or the practice of yoga.If at all if there is reason our birth, there has been always a purpose to be fullled in your life, and if at all that happens it adds beauty to your life and a meaning in your death!!

WHY DO YOGIS SAY NAMASTE

Probably if you have been to any yoga class, you would have seen yogic instructors or practitioners bowing and saying "Namaste" at the beginning of the class. In India this gesture is common and understood.But many of us actually do this without knowing it's proper meaning and the purpose. May sound simple but many of us still don't know why we do that.When asked about it they say, I did it because everyone were doing the same. It's like a flock of sheep following the shepherd.The sheeps never know the way but just go behind the shepherd.

To understand the meaning of Namaste we have to break down the word into three parts. The rst word "Namah" tells us to bow or respectful salutation. The second word "As" translates to "I" and the last word "Te" means "to you".Overall it means "I bow down to you".As said earlier every individual has a divine being or soul within himself. So the divine in me bows down to the divine in you. We always should understand that we all are a part of this creation. Once you bow down, the likes and dislikes in you diminishes and the process of "oneness" with the creation arises within you. This is the intention behind doing namaskar. Yoga always says that there is a source of creation for every cell and atom in this universe. That source of creation resides deep within you. This is why in Indian culture, if you looked up at the sky, the culture taught you to bow down. If you look down at the earth, you bow down. If you see a man, a woman, a child, a cow, a tree or whatever, you bow down. And it is a constant reminder that the source of creation is within you too. Hence you bring both your palms together in ashwini mudra and bow down and greet with namaskar.If I want to say in a normal sense, taking out of philosophy behind it, namaste always means bowing down to the truth and wisdom that lies in the heart of other. Whoever it be, every part of that creation has some beauty and wisdom embedded in it nomatter how much ever wicked the person is, we can always learn something from every being in the universe. As Swami Vivekananda says, “Each soul is potentially divine”. Namaste is often accompanied with the hands pressed together in prayer position at the heart and a slight bow is given. This is also a beautiful moment for us to express love from our heart and humility. But in India this way of greeting people is always seen down and people always feel comfortable in greeting by shaking hands and hugging each other with words “hello”, " hi" as such. We must always be aware that our age old tradition of greeting with Namaste along with philosophy had also a science behind it that was thought by our ancestors. There is a scientific reason behind the ‘Namaskar’ in Hindu culture. Joining both hands ensures touching the tips of all the fingers together, which are linked to pressure points in the eyes, ears, and mind. Pressing them together is said to activate these, helping us remember that person for a long time and also Namaste done unintentionally activates all the very important nerve endings and vital points in the palms. This is a very beneficial therapeutic practice that can tone up several body systems and balance several inconsistencies and hormonal secretions in the body.The gesture of namaste is unique also in the sense that its physical performance is accompanied by a verbal utterance of the word "namaste." This practice is equivalent to the chanting of a mantra. The sonority of the sacred sound 'namaste' is believed to have a magical value, corresponding to a creative energy change. This transformation is that of aligning oneself in harmony with the vibration of the other.So now moving on further nowadays we all are aware that this Indian practice of performing namaskar is being appreciated and followed by the western people. The rampant spread of corona virus and huge death toll has triggered alarms in the world community. We all are re-evaluating our customs, beliefs, food habits through which the disease can be spread. One such concern is the way we greet. In recent times, Centre for Disease Centre for Disease Control and Prevention alerted that shaking hands can be a cause for transmission of Corona virus. Hence people have now started reinventing and recommending the several other benefits of Namaste, the Indian traditional way of greeting that does not involve any physical contact with the other person. When the whole world is attracted towards Indian tradition and practices, it's our prime duty to uphold our culture and tradition for it is the one which makes India stand firmly and strongly apart from rest of the world. So let's always start this practice of greeting everyone with "Namaste" not just in our yoga class but also in our day to day lives!!

www.ingramcontent.com/pod-product-compliance
Lightning Source LLC
LaVergne TN
LVHW050407160726
843469LV00041B/987

* 9 7 8 9 3 5 6 1 0 5 7 6 8 *